MILADY'S
STANDARD
COSMETOLOGY

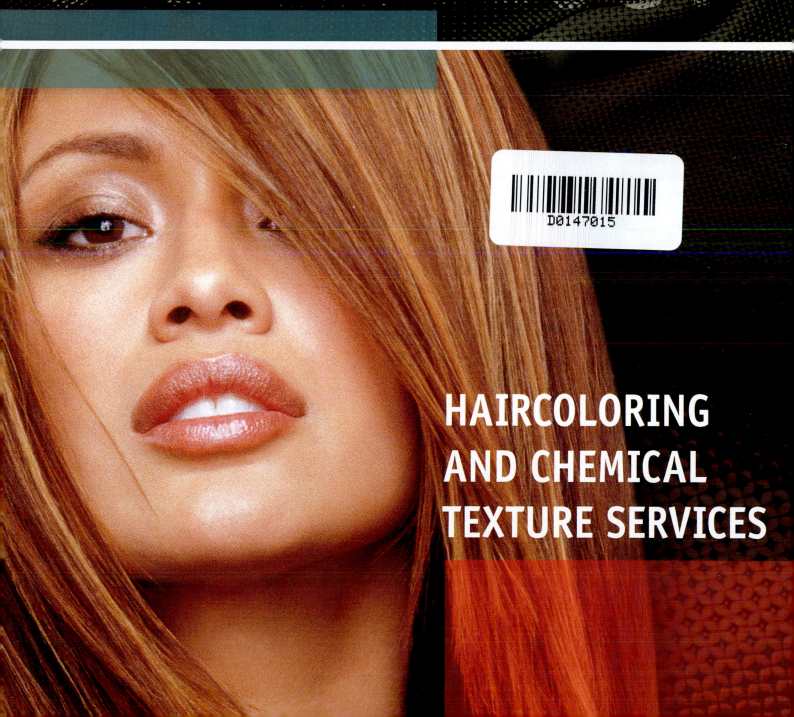

HAIRCOLORING
AND CHEMICAL
TEXTURE SERVICES

MILADY'S
STANDARD
COSMETOLOGY

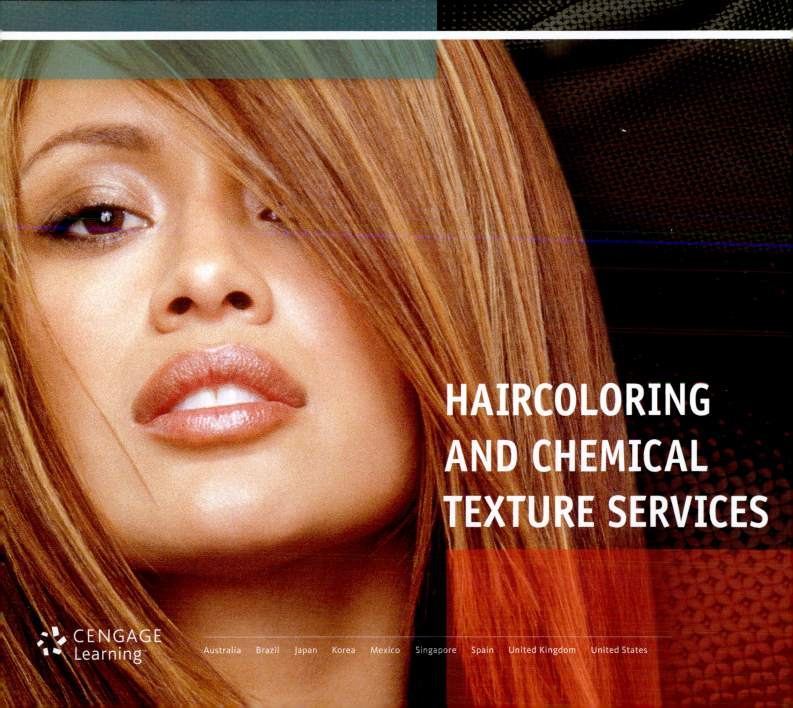

HAIRCOLORING
AND CHEMICAL
TEXTURE SERVICES

CENGAGE
Learning

Australia   Brazil   Japan   Korea   Mexico   Singapore   Spain   United Kingdom   United States

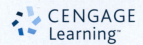

**Milady's Standard Cosmetology:
Hair coloring and Chemical Texturing
Services, First Edition**
Milady

President, Milady: Dawn Gerrain

Publisher: Erin O'Connor

Product Manager: Jessica Burns

Editorial Assistant: Maria Hebert

Director of Beauty Industry Relations:
  Sandra Bruce

Senior Marketing Manager: Gerard McAvey

Production Director: Wendy Troeger

Senior Content Project Manager:
  Nina Tucciarelli

Senior Art Director: Joy Kocsis

For product information and technology assistance, contact us at
Professional & Career Group Customer Support, 1-800-648-7450

For permission to use material from this text or product,
submit all requests online at **cengage.com/permissions**
Further permissions questions can be emailed to
permissionrequest@cengage.com

Library of Congress Control Number: 2009910819

ISBN-13: 978-1-1110-3615-7

ISBN-10: 1-1110-3615-2

Milady
5 Maxwell Drive
Clifton Park, NY 12065-2919
USA

Cengage Learning products are represented in Canada by Nelson Education, Ltd.

For your lifelong learning solutions, visit **milady.cengage.com**

Visit our corporate website at **cengage.com**

Notice to the Reader
Publisher does not warrant or guarantee any of the products described herein or perform any independent analysis in connection with any of the product information contained herein. Publisher does not assume, and expressly disclaims, any obligation to obtain and include information other than that provided to it by the manufacturer. The reader is expressly warned to consider and adopt all safety precautions that might be indicated by the activities described herein and to avoid all potential hazards. By following the instructions contained herein, the reader willingly assumes all risks in connection with such instructions. The publisher makes no representations or warranties of any kind, including but not limited to, the warranties of fitness for particular purpose or merchantability, nor are any such representations implied with respect to the material set forth herein, and the publisher takes no responsibility with respect to such material. The publisher shall not be liable for any special, consequential, or exemplary damages resulting, in whole or part, from the readers' use of, or reliance upon, this material.

Printed in China
3 4 5 6 7 14 13 12 11

TABLE OF CONTENTS

PREFACE

vii

Milady's Standard Cosmetology: Haircoloring and Chemical Texture Services is a new, full-color, spiral bound supplement to the leading cosmetology textbook *Milady's Standard Cosmetology*. This book provides you with step-by-step technicals for haircoloring and chemical texture services. Each technical features two categories, an overview and an apply. The overview is a short introduction providing a framework about the techniques you will learn. The "apply" is the step-by-step part of the technique. Each step is explained in detail and is accompanied throughout by photos. Many of the techniques will also have a Variation of the technique. Each technique will end with photos of the same technique performed on different hair lengths, colors and textures to help ignite your imagination. This will help you consider different possibilities to applying what you've learned in many creative ways.

IMAGE CREDITS

Photography by Tom Carson and glamour photos courtesy of the following salons:

- Glynn Jones Salon, Alexandria, VA
- Carmen Carmen Salon & Spa, Charlotte, NC
- Bob Steele Salon, Atlanta, GA
- Steele Salon, Atlanta, GA
- Ladies & Gentlemen Salon & Spa, Mentor, OH
- John Roberts Salon & Spa, Cleveland, OH
- PSC, Chicago, IL
- The Brown Aveda Institute, Mentor, OH
- Ladies & Gentlemen Salon & Spa, Mentor, OH
- Salon Exclusive

HAIRCOLORING

 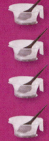
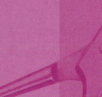

PATCH TEST

OVERVIEW

The most important part of the client consultation is to find out all you can about her. Take down necessary information so that you can always have it on record. When working with chemicals such as haircolor, you will have to find out if the client has any sensitivities or allergic reactions to anything. Use the patch test on a client who has never had a haircolor service to see if she has any reaction.

APPLY

ON DVD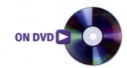

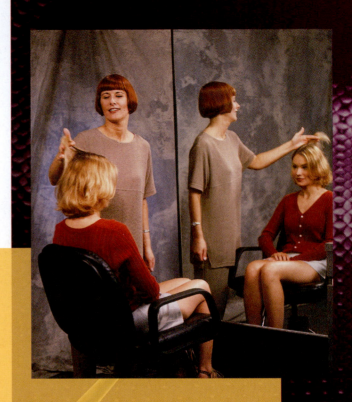

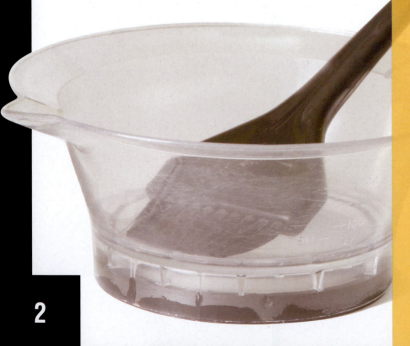

PROCEDURE

1. Explain to your client that this test must be done to see if she has any sensitivities to color.

2. Determine the product for the haircolor service.

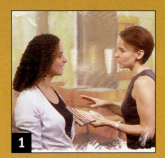 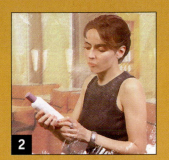

3. Mix a small amount of the product in a bowl.

4. Apply it to the inside of your client's elbow with a cotton swab.

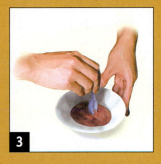 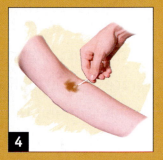

5. Let the color dry.

6. Examine the results in 24 hours. If there is no irritation on the area, you can move forward with the service.

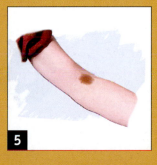 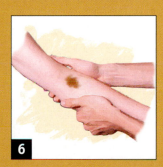

STRAND TEST

OVERVIEW

Now that you have learned the different categories of haircolor products, along with the different characteristics of hair, you are ready to begin strand testing. This is the most important part of the haircolor process. It establishes what the haircolor result is going to look like. The strand test is especially vital when working with new clients or clients with chemically challenged hair.

APPLY

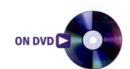 ON DVD ▶

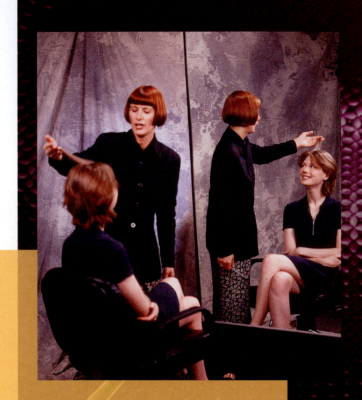

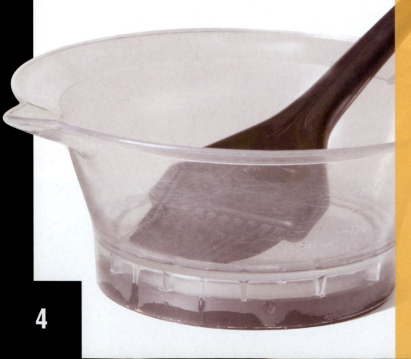

PROCEDURE

1. During the client consultation, explain why it is necessary to strand test the hair before starting.

2. Determine and mix the formula.

3. Apply the formula underneath a strand of hair in the back of the head. Wrap that piece of hair in foil.

4. Set a timer for 10 minutes.

5. After the timer goes off, wipe the area using a water bottle and a towel.

6. Check the resulting color development.

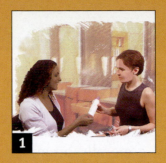

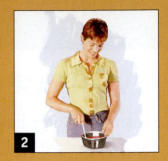

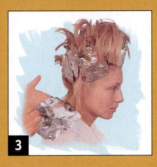

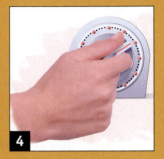

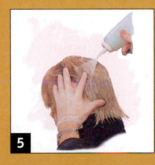

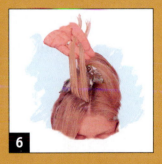

MIXING

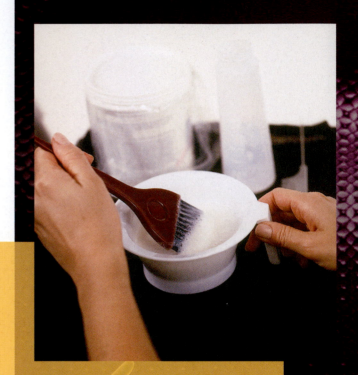

OVERVIEW

Learning to mix haircolor is a very important skill. It will generally be mixed in equal proportion (1:1), or two to one (2:1), meaning two parts developer to one part color. (This is most often a high-lift blonde formula.) Most of these products combine a color and a developer. Most are mixed in equal proportions, although some are not. Lighteners are mixed differently from color products. In the steps below, you'll mix combinations of different products.

APPLY

ON DVD ▶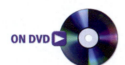

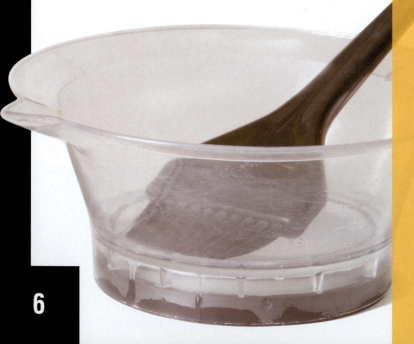

PROCEDURE

Applicator Bottle (1:1 Mixing)

1. Pour 2 oz. of the developer into the applicator bottle.

2. Add 2 oz. of the color.

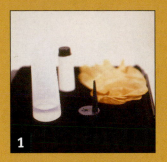
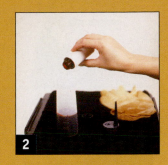

3. Put the top on the bottle and shake gently until mixed.

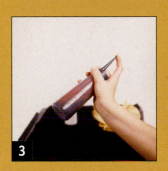

Applicator Bottle (2:1 Mixing)

1. Here, 2:1 mixing is shown for a high-lift blonde color formula. Pour 4 oz. of developer into the applicator bottle.

2. Add 2 oz. of color into the bottle. Use all contents in the 2 oz. tube of cream color.

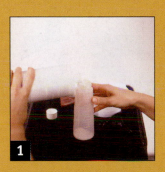
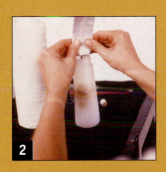

3. Put the top on the bottle and mix gently and thoroughly.

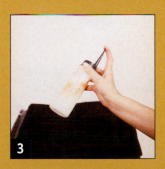

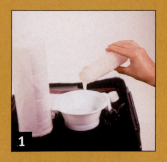 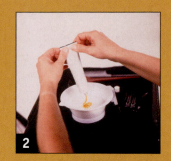

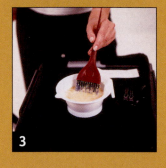

Bowl and Brush (1:1 Mixing)

1. Pour 2 oz. of developer into an applicator bottle. Pour the developer into bowl.

2. Squeeze 2 oz. of color into the bowl.

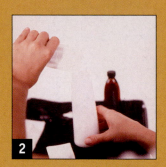

3. Mix to a creamy consistency.

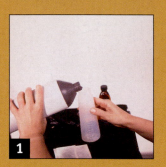 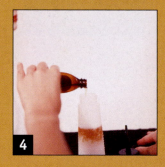

On-the-Scalp Lighteners (2:1 Mixing)

1. Pour 4 oz. of 20-volume developer into the applicator bottle.

2. Add one to three lightening activators according to the amount of lightening desired. Follow the manufacturer directions.

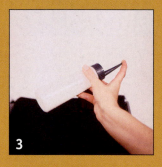

3. Put the top on the bottle and shake gently.

4. Add 2 oz. of lightener to the bottle.

5. Put the top on the bottle and shake gently.

Off-the-Scalp Powder Lighteners

1. To mix off-the-scalp powder lighteners, pour 2 ½ oz. of developer into a nonmetallic bowl.

2. Add 4 scoops of powder lightener to the bowl.

3. Mix to creamy consistency.

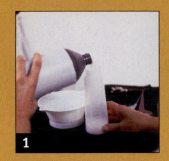
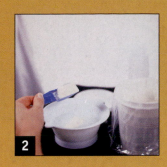

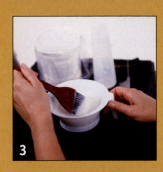

COLOR ENHANCEMENT FOR RELAXED HAIR

OVERVIEW

Color enhancement is a great way to introduce a client to color services. Enhancements add tone and shine in one easy step to any haircolor—without lightening the hair. A color enhancement may complement a wide variety of hair types, whether blonde, red, brunette, or black hair. The total color service takes about 20 minutes. In the following steps you will enhance the color of brunette hair, both textured and relaxed.

Mastering color enhancements will build a strong foundation for other haircolor situations you will encounter. Learning good formulation and application skills is very important.

APPLY

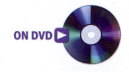

ON DVD ▶

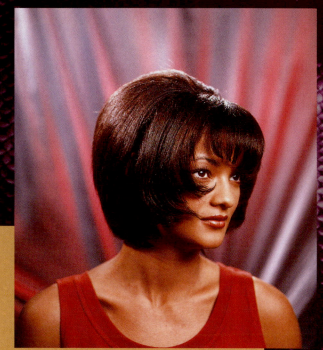

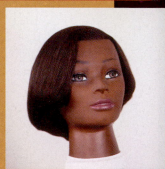

PROCEDURE

1. Mix the formula, using 1:1 proportions of 2 oz. Medium Red Brown with 2 oz. of demi-permanent developer. Wear gloves when you mix and apply color. Section the hair with the tip of the applicator bottle.

2. Outline the hair into four sections—from ear to ear and from front forehead to center nape.

3. Begin applying where it is determined that the hair is the most resistant. Here, you'll start in the front right section. Take ½" partings and apply the color to the base area, working neatly, precisely, and efficiently. Bring all sections out away from the head to allow air to circulate. Move to the front left section and apply color to the base area, again taking ½" partings. Continue until the section is complete.

4. Move onto the back sections of the head, following the same method. Work neatly until this section is completed.

5. After all four sections have color on the base area, work the color down the hair shaft to the ends, making sure the hair is saturated with color. Gently massage the color through all of the hair. Do not rub or work aggressively. Set the timer for up to 20 minutes to process the color.

6. Previously drab in tone; now note how the rich color accentuates this relaxed hair. Coloring and relaxing services can both be done successfully on the same day with non-ammonia, color-enhancing products.

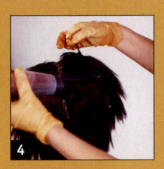

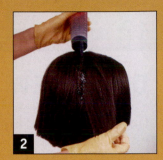

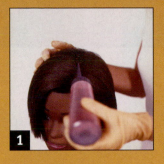

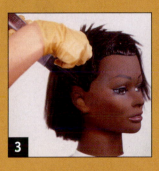

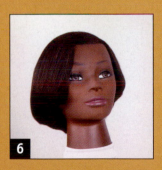

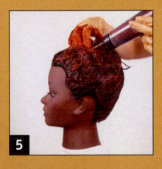

VARIATION—COLOR ENHANCEMENT ON TEXTURED HAIR

OVERVIEW

On this, the Textured Light Layered Shape, a color enhancement formula is used to add rich warmth and dimension to the hair.

APPLY

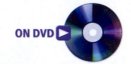 ON DVD

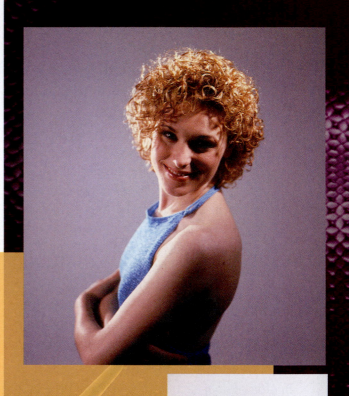

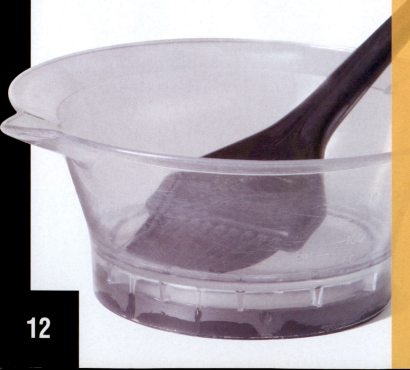

PROCEDURE

1. Mix the formula, using 2 oz. of 6R Dark Red Blonde and 2 oz. of demi-permanent developer. Wear gloves when you mix and apply color. Section the hair with the tip of the applicator bottle.

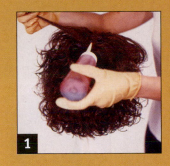

2. Outline the hair into four sections from ear to ear and from front forehead to center nape. After all sections have color on the base area, work the color down the hair shaft to the ends, making sure the hair is saturated with color. Gently massage the color through the hair. Do not rub or work aggressively. Set the time for up to 20 minutes to process the color. Remember to shorten the processing time for porous hair.

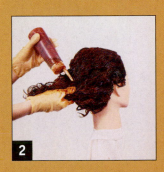

3. The finished color adds richness and dimension to the textured hair. Coloring and texture services can be done successfully on the same day with non-ammonia, color-enhancing products.

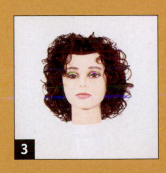

CREATE

Apply this technique to different hair lengths, colors, and cuts for almost endless possibilities.

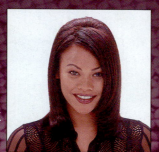 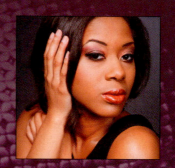 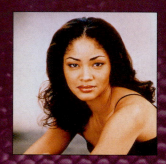

PERMANENT HAIRCOLOR: PHASE 1—VIRGIN APPLICATIONS

OVERVIEW

Now that you have worked with non-ammonia color-enhancing products, it is time to graduate to the next phase of haircolor: permanent haircolor. This can lighten natural color, change tone, and cover gray hair—the possibilities are endless.

You will begin permanent haircoloring by lightening natural pigment. This is referred to as a *virgin application going lighter*. It is a popular service with clients who want to lighten and change the tone of their existing color.

APPLY

ON DVD ▶

The graduated blunt cut will be dramatically transformed with the application of permanent color throughout all of the hair. The deep brunette color will be lightened to a warm red-brown.

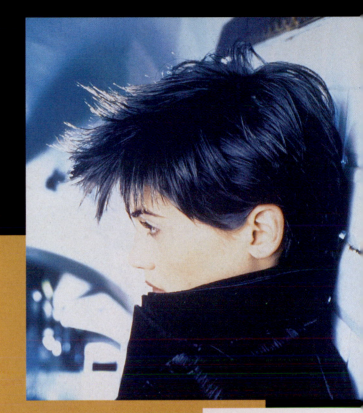
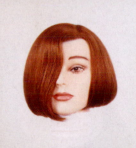
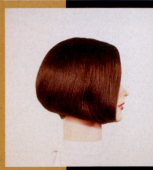

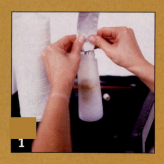
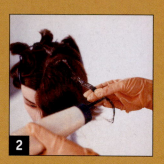

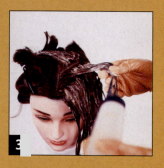
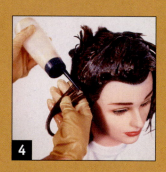

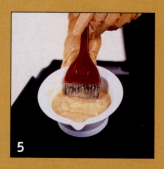
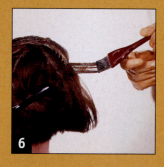

PROCEDURE

1. Mix the formula—pour 4 oz. of 20 volume developer in first, then add the color, 20 of 12 Lightest Golden Blonde.

2. Divide the hair into four sections—from ear to ear and straight down the back of the head. Take a ½" subsection beginning in the top area of the head, then apply the product ½" away from the scalp and work down to the ends.

3. Working down the section, apply the color ½" away from the scalp. Work it through to the midshaft and then to the ends.

4. Continue around the head with the same application technique. Note how the tip of the applicator bottle is multi-purpose in that it neatly parts out the ½" sections, then dispenses the product on the hair, as well as spreads the product along the length of the hair.

5. For illustrative purposes, the images here show a bowl and brush will be used to apply through the back area of the head. Mix the formula following the manufacturer's directions.

6. Apply the color to the back of the head taking ½" subsections and applying ½" away from the scalp.

7. Work precisely and quickly through each section. Use the brush and the fingers to work the color formula into the hair.

8. Next, complete the fourth quadrant.

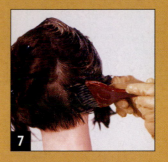
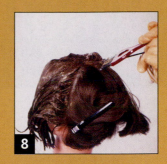

9. Continue the application process down to the nape hairline area. Where lengths are extremely short in this area, work color throughout.

10. Set the time for 25 minutes.

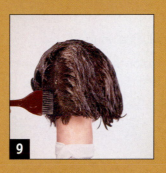
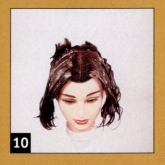

11. Apply the color to the base area in all four sections. Outline the quadrants first.

12. Take ½" subsections, working through each one until the head is completed. Work neatly and efficiently, dispensing color along the base area and then working in with the applicator bottle tip. Part out each new parting and dispense the color along the upper part of the parting as shown. Make sure to apply enough color to thoroughly saturate the hair, including around the front hairline.

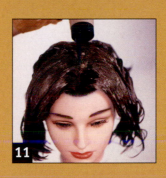
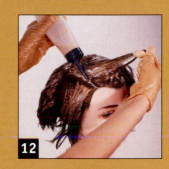

13. Work through the interior of the back quadrants using the brush method introduced earlier.

14. Set the timer for an additional 20 minutes. The total processing time is 45 minutes.

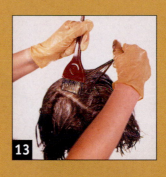
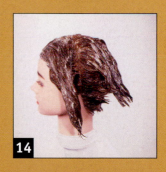

15. This permanent color change lightens brunette hair to a warmer brown with soft red tones.

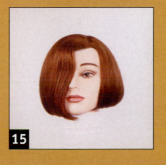

17

APPLY

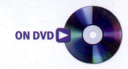

ON DVD ▶

PROCEDURE

1. Greet the client by introducing yourself.

2. Discuss the type of hair color the client is looking for. Mix 1 oz. 3RV Medium Red Violet Brown, 1 oz. Light Red Orange Brown, and 2 oz. 20 volume developer.

3. Using the tip of an applicator bottle, divide the hair into four sections.

4. Apply the color ½" away from the scalp to outline the four sections.

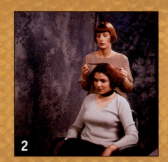
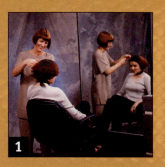
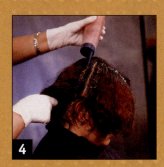
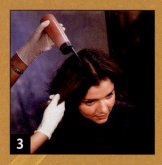
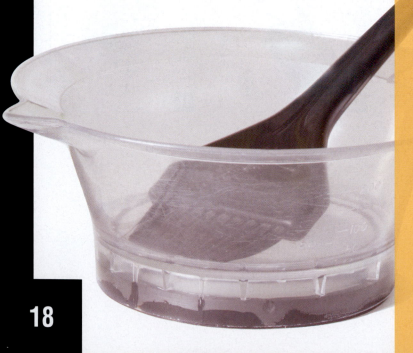

5. Start at the right front section and apply the color ½" away from the scalp. It is a good idea to always start the application in the front sections of the head, to obtain maximum coverage through the front areas.

6. Take ½" subsections and continue applying color ½" from the scalp area down the hair strand.

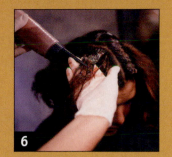
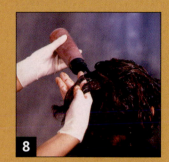

7. Develop a rhythm of speed in working to get the product on the entire head as quickly as possible. Thoroughly saturate each section of hair for thorough coverage.

8. Continue around the head until all four sections are complete.

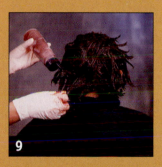
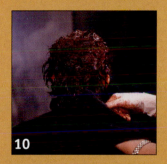

9. Set the timer for 25 minutes. Next, apply color to the base area. Work around the outline first, then work into the interior of each section.

10. Continue applying color to the base area around the entire head. Work the color through the hair and set the timer for 20 minutes. Rinse. Shampoo and condition. Style and finish hair.

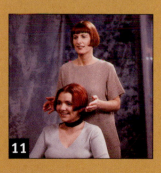
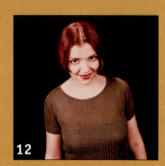

11. Check the color, record the color formula, and recommend home maintenance.

12. The finished look is a vivid high-fashion red.

CREATE

Apply this technique to different hair lengths, colors, and cuts for almost endless possibilities.

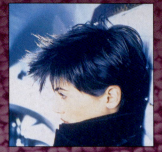
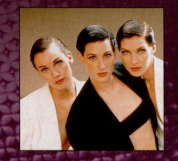
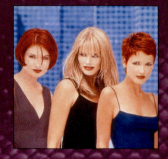
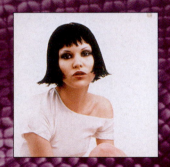
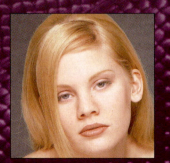
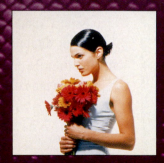

PERMANENT HAIRCOLOR: PHASE 2—SINGLE-PROCESS RETOUCH WITH A GLAZE

OVERVIEW

Once a client has had a color application, her next visit will involve a retouch. This means you will use permanent haircolor only to lighten the new growth at the scalp area. To refresh the ends, you will formulate a non-ammonia color that adds shine and tone to the hair without lightening it. This technique is proven to keep the hair in the best condition with minimal fading—because you do not use permanent color, which has ammonia, down the shaft and on the ends of the hair.

You have already learned how to use non-ammonia color and permanent haircolor products. Now you will use them both on the same head. This is called a single-process retouch with a glaze. It is the most sophisticated way to use permanent color. In a retouch application, you apply permanent color only to the new growth of the hair.

Formulate the color referring to the color chart. The color generally needs to process 45 minutes. After rinsing and towel drying, the glaze will be applied through the lengths.

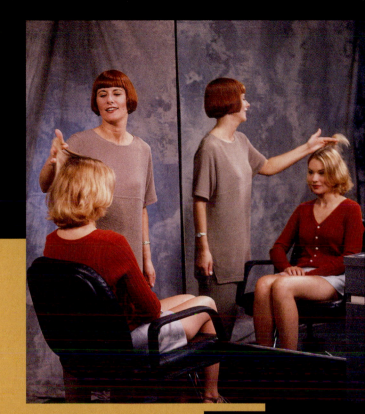

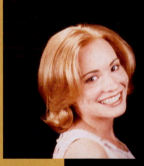

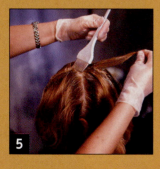

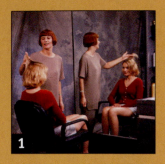

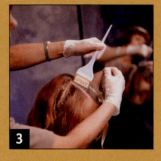

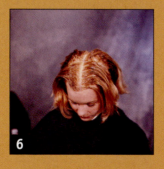

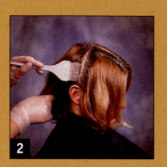

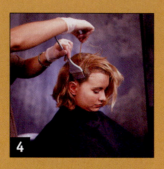

APPLY

ON DVD ▶

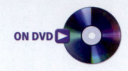

PROCEDURE

1. Greet your client by introducing yourself. In consultation, discuss the haircolor results she is looking for. Mix the formula. Apply a high-lift blonde formula at the retouch area first—2 oz. of 12G Lightest Golden Blonde and 4 oz. of 40 volume developer.

2. Using a color brush, begin by outlining all four sections of the regrowth. Then apply color to the regrowth area within each quadrant.

3. Starting at the front right section, apply the color with the color brush to the new growth at the base area.

4. Continue working down the right side, taking ¼″ subsections and applying the color to the new growth.

5. Continue around the head taking fine, even sections.

6. Complete all four sides. Set the timer for 45 minutes. When the time is up, rinse the color thoroughly.

7. Mix the glaze—1 ½ oz. of 10RO, Red-Orange Blonde, ½ oz. 8G, Light Golden Blonde, and 2 oz. of demi-permanent developer. Now it is time to apply the non-ammonia haircolor glaze. Start at the front hairline.

8. Apply the glaze in a base-to-ends fashion, moving it through the hair quickly. Set the time for up to 15 minutes. Rinse. Shampoo and condition.

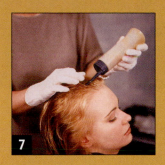

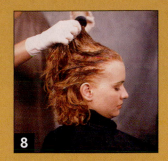

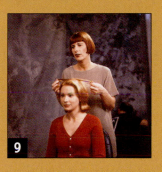

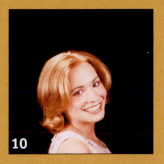

9. Check hair color results, and recommend home maintenance to your client.

10. Here is the finished look: a light, warm blonde color that is even from the base to ends, with lots of vibrant shine.

CREATE

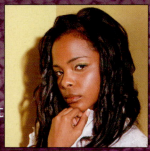

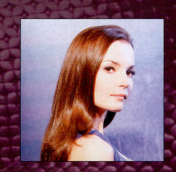

Apply this technique to different hair lengths, colors, and cuts for almost endless possibilities.

PERMANENT HAIRCOLOR: PHASE 3—COVERING GRAY

OVERVIEW

Gray hair is still the number one reason why people color their hair. To cover gray completely, your best choice is a permanent haircolor—but there are different ways to change gray hair to suit the client. Understanding the difference between blending and covering is key to a successful consultation. When a client sees that he is faced with a few gray hairs, he usually want to get rid of them. He will say things like, "Can I try a color?" or, "Can I make the gray hair look highlighted?" This is when you should reach for a non-ammonia color to blend the gray. This type of color service has more sheer results, and it will also wash out faster, meaning it is less permanent. Once the client starts seeing more than just a few gray hairs, however, he is usually looking to get rid of them completely. Now you should reach for a permanent color to cover the gray.

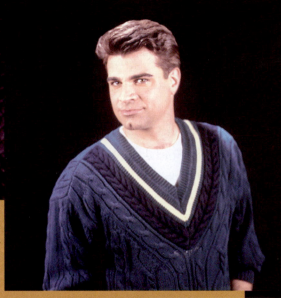

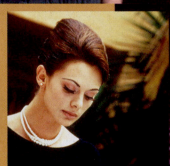

APPLY

ON DVD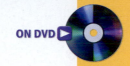

PROCEDURE

1. Introduce yourself to the client. Discuss the color results that he is looking for. The formula to be used is 1 oz. of Dark Natural Blonde, 1 oz. of Light Golden Brown, and 2 oz. of 20 volume developer.

2. Start the application down the front center part. Apply the color to the base area only.

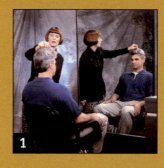

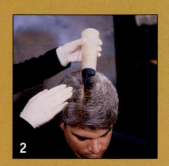

3. Part out ¼" subsections and apply the color to the base area.

4. Continue around the head using ¼" subsections.

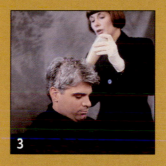

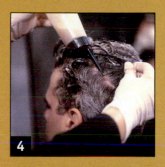

5. Once all four sections are complete, work the rest of the color through to the ends. Process the color for 45 minutes.

6. Record all formulas and recommended specific shampoos and conditioners for color-treated hair. Notice how one simple formula can make a client look more youthful.

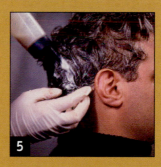

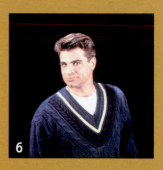

CREATE

Apply this technique to different hair lengths, colors, and cuts for almost endless possibilities.

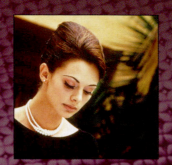

DOUBLE-PROCESS BLONDING

OVERVIEW

There are different ways to make hair blonde. To create the lightest blonde all over the head, especially on clients who have dark hair to start with, a double-process is best. This involves two steps: lightening the hair, and then toning the hair.

In this segment you will learn to identify how lighteners react on the hair. In addition, once the hair has been lightened, it must be toned. In this lightening process, you will first remove all natural pigment from the hair with an on-the-scalp lightener. This haircolor service is for the client who wants to be the blondest she can be.

APPLY

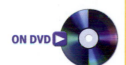
ON DVD

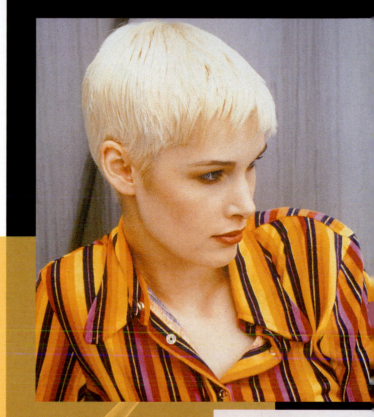

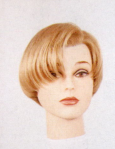

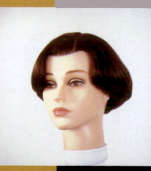

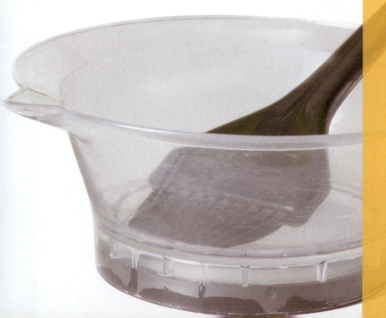

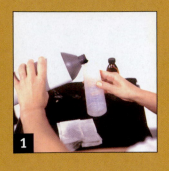

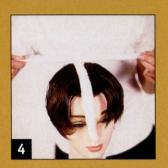

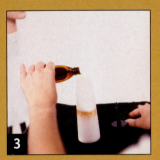

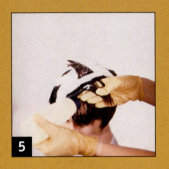

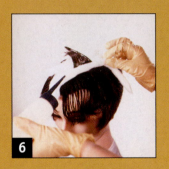

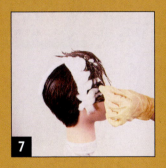

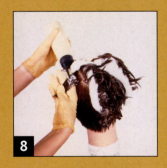

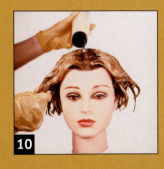

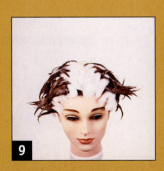

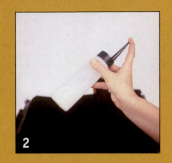

PROCEDURE

1. Pour 4 oz. of 20 volume peroxide into a bottle. Add up to three lightening activators, also called catalysts.

2. Shake gently until mixed.

3. Add 2 oz. of liquid lightener.

4. Place cotton in all four quadrants to protect the scalp. (This is an option that may or may not be used.)

5. Starting in the left front section, apply lightener ¼" away from the scalp. Work it down through to the ends with the gloved hand.

6. Place a strip of cotton in between each section so that no lightener bleeds onto the hair nearest the scalp.

7. Take ¼" sections and work until the side is complete.

8. Through the back, the technique of application will be shown without cotton strips. Continue ¼" sections starting ½" away from the scalp, working the lightener down the ends.

9. Complete all four sections, and set the timer for 25 minutes.

10. After the 25 minutes are up, remove the cotton. Start applying the lightener to the base area.

11. Continue to apply the lightener to the base area within the interior area of all sections.

12. After all sections are complete, work the rest of the lightener through the hair so it is completely saturated. Set the timer for 30 minutes.

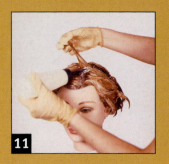
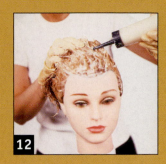

13. Do a strand test to check for desired lightness. Place a strand on a white towel, then spray with a water bottle to remove the lightener. When complete, rinse and shampoo. Now you are ready to apply the toner.

14. Lightened hair should be handled delicately. Towel dry the hair thoroughly. Be gentle to the hair as you divide it into four quadrants. Begin outlining with the toner mixture—2 oz 8N Light Neutral Blonde and 2 oz of demi-permanent developer. Hair that has just been lightened is fragile.

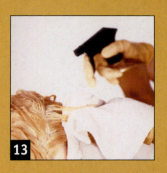
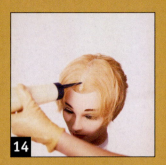

15. Starting at the front, apply the toner to the base area.

16. Continue moving quickly around the head.

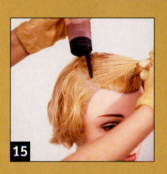
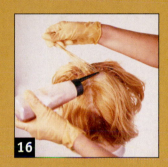

17. Set the timer for five minutes.

18. After the five minutes are up, start working the remainder of the toner down to the ends.

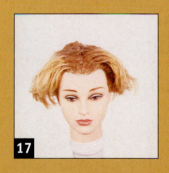
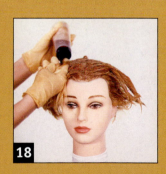

19. Let the toner process for another five to ten minutes. Complete a strand test to see if the color result is there.

20. What a dramatic transformation—from the Level 3 (Dark Brown) to this dramatic blonde tone! This is the clarity you can create with a double-process blonding.

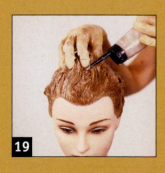
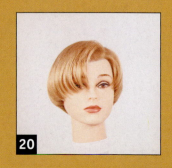

CREATE

Apply this technique to different hair lengths, colors, and cuts for almost endless possibilities.

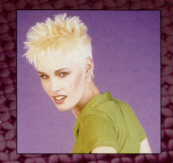

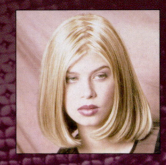

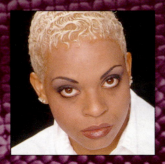

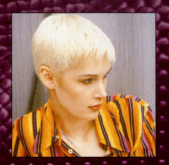

DIMENSIONAL HAIRCOLOR SERVICES

OVERVIEW

Dimensional haircolor services—better known as highlighting—are one of the fastest-growing haircolor markets. This is where your creativity is endless. Foiling is the professional choice for highlighting the hair. It provides tremendous control in the application, and creates precision results. Here you will learn some of the most popular techniques used in the salon today. We will focus on four different foil-wrapping methods: face frame highlight, three-quarter head highlight, and full head highlight. The specific application process may be recorded to ensure that you reproduce results on the client's next visit.

FACE FRAME HIGHLIGHTS

APPLY

ON DVD ▶

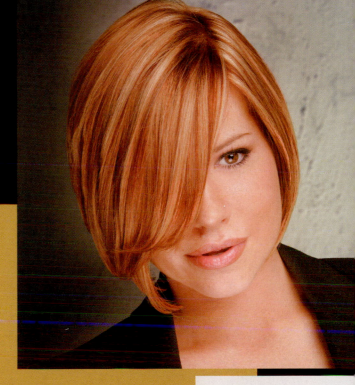

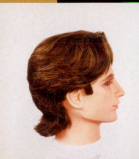

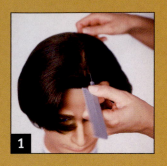

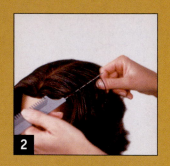

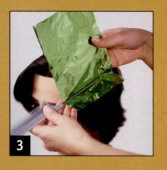

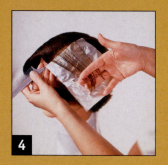

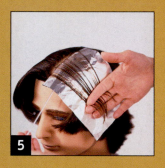

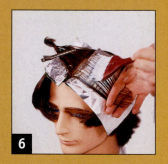

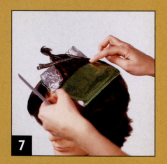

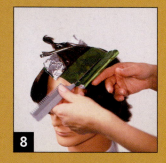

PROCEDURE

1. With a tail or foil-tip comb, part the hair from ear to ear, with a part going down the center.

2. Starting at the center part, part out ⅛" slice with the tail end of your comb.

3. While holding the slice of hair, pick up a piece of foil. Fold the end of the comb under the foil and place it at the scalp.

4. Lay the hair on top of the foil, getting as close to the scalp as possible.

5. Slide the comb out from underneath. Hold hair taut to the foil.

6. Brush on lightener, starting ½" away from the top of the foil and working the product down the strand. Once the product adheres to the hair in the foil, work it up to the top of the foil.

7. Fold the foil in half to meet the piece at the top.

8. With the metal end of your comb, crease the center of the foil.

9. Fold the foil again and slide the metal end of your comb out.

10. Clip the foil up and out of the way.

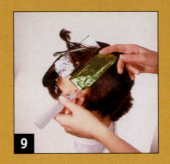 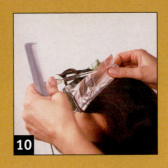

11. Part out ½" subsection of hair in between each foiled slide.

12. Clip each foil section up and out of the way.

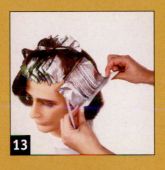 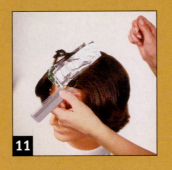

13. Continue working down the side in the same way. The foils on the side will go to the temple area. Once one side is complete, move to the other.

14. Here, all the foils are in.

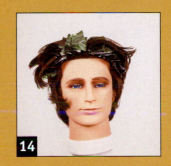 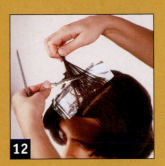

15. Open a foil to see if the color has reached the desired lightness. When complete, rinse thoroughly, then shampoo and condition. Apply a glaze if desired.

16. Notice how this service adds a subtle amount of dimension that frames the face.

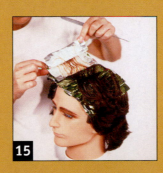 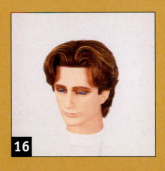

HALF-HEAD HIGHLIGHT

In this service, you will highlight the top and sides of the head.

APPLY

ON DVD ▶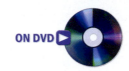

PROCEDURE

1. Block off sections. The three main sections are the top and the sides. Take a fine ⅛" slice starting at the crown of the head.

2. While holding the slice of hair, pick up a piece of foil. Fold the end of the comb under the foil and place it at the scalp.

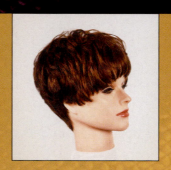
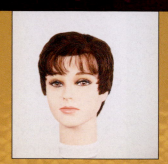

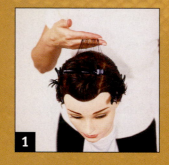
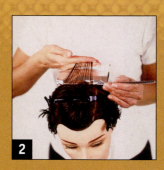

3. Brush on lightener, starting ½" away from the top of the foil, working the product down the strand. Double fold the foil.

4. Release the next ½" section and clip out of the way. Continue working toward the front of the head.

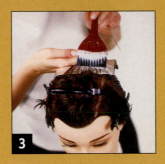
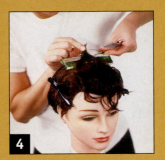

5. To create a chunk look toward the front, take the metal end of your comb and weave it back and forth through the strand.

6. Slide your comb from underneath the foil. Notice the hair in the foil.

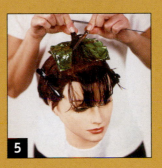
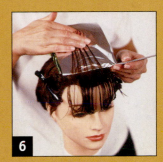

7. Apply the product to the hair.

8. Bend the foil once over the hair, and then fold the foil again. Fold the foil and clip it out of the way.

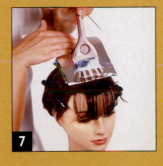
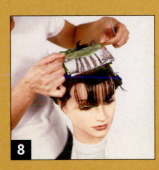

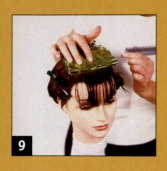

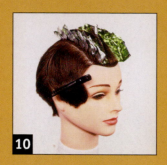

9. Part out an approximately ½" section to leave unfoiled, then part out a ⅛" section for the next foil. Complete up to the front hairline.

10. The top of the head is complete. It is now time to do the sides.

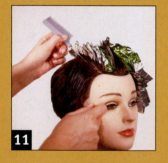

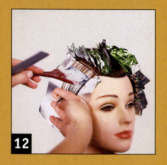

11. Take a fine ⅛" slice at the top section of the right side.

12. After placing the foil, apply the product, working down the entire strand.

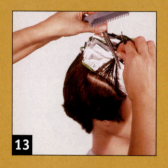

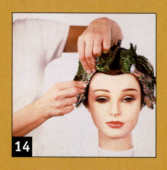

13. Clip the foil up and out of the way. Clip a section out of the way to go unlightened between each foil.

14. Complete both sides.

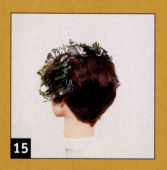

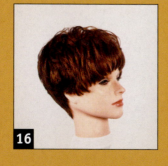

15. This half-head technique covers the entire front portion of the head.

16. This haircolor technique adds dimension that covers a fairly wide surface of the head.

THREE-QUARTER HEAD HIGHLIGHT

In this service, you will provide highlights over the entire head, all the way down to the occipital bone in the back.

APPLY

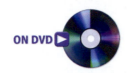

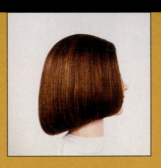

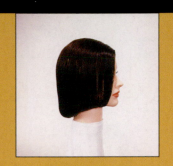

PROCEDURE

1. After blocking off the head into six sections or panels, start at the center back crown area. Part out a fine slice, place the foil as shown, and apply the lightener. Enclose the hair with a double-fold method. Clip the hair up and out of the way.

2. Take ½" subsections between each foil. Clip these sections up and out of the way.

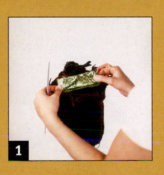

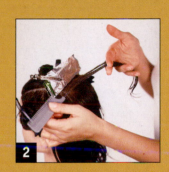

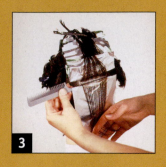

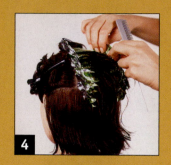

3. Continue placing the foils down to the occipital bone using the procedure as outlined. Upon completion, release all the clipped up foils. Turn the edges of the foil on either side.

4. Here is the completed back section.

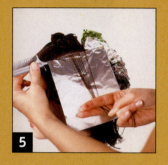

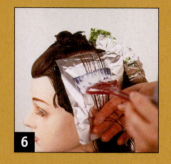

5. Move to a side section. You'll place these foils with a book end method. Take a fine slice. Place hair in the center third of the foil.

6. Apply the product to the hair in the foil.

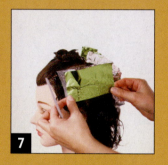

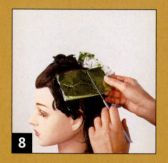

7. Fold the foil in half until the ends meet.

8. Fold the right side of the foil in halfway, using your comb to crease it.

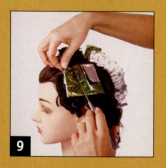

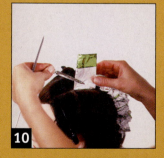

9. Fold the left side of the foil in halfway.

10. Clip the foil upward. Notice the book-wrap effect.

11. Take a ½" subsection in between the foils.

12. Continue working down the back side until you reach the occipital area. Complete this section on the opposite side.

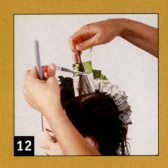

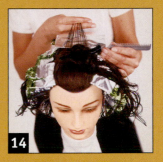

13. Move to the front sections and continue foiling. Use the same technique as outlined.

14. After completing both sides, continue wrapping the top portion of the head, taking ½" subsections in between the foils. Alternate the process of fine slices with ½" slices left unfoiled.

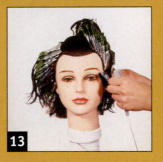

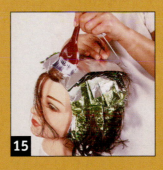

15. Finish the last foil at the hairline. Fold the sides of the foil up on each side to secure them in place.

16. This finished look gives a very desirable and natural dimensional effect throughout, accentuated further by the unlightened nape area. Apply a toner to create a harmonious blend of highlights to natural hair.

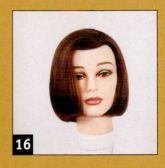

FULL-HEAD HIGHLIGHT

Highlights all over the head give the brightest look to a client.

APPLY

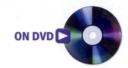
ON DVD ▶

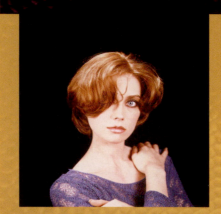

PROCEDURE

1. Consult with your client regarding her hair color wishes.
2. Take a slice of hair at the lower crown area of the head.

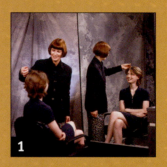

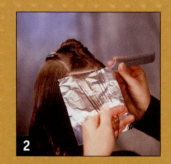

3. Holding the hair taut, brush lightener onto the hair in the foil.
4. Double fold the foil and clip up and out of the way.

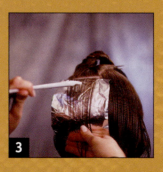

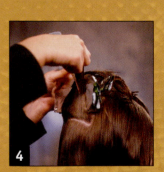

5. Take a ¾" subsection in between the foils.

6. Continue working down the back center of the head until the section is complete. Note the contrast in size between the foiled and unfoiled sections.

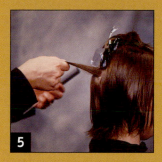 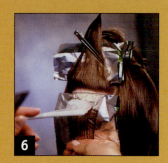

7. Once the section is complete, release the clipped-up foil.

8. Working around the head, into the side area, divide the panel into two smaller sections.

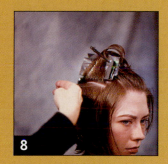 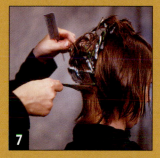

9. Continue working down the side by taking fine slices of hair into the foil. Continue through the center back. Clip everything up and out of the way.

10. Move to the other side of the head and complete this same panel.

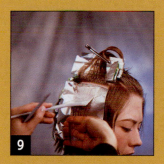 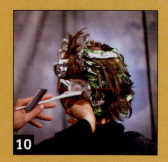

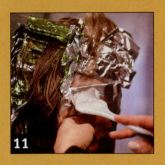

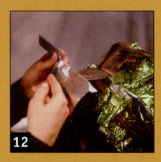

11. Finish the front panels on each side of the head with the same method.

12. Now it is time to do the last section—the top of the head. Take a fine slice of hair off the top of a larger section and place it on the foil.

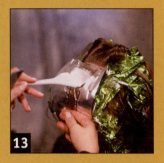

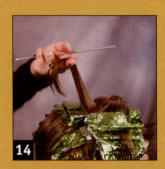

13. Apply the product to the hair.

14. Part out a larger section, and then take a fine slice from the top of this section.

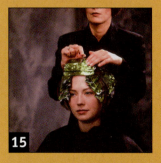

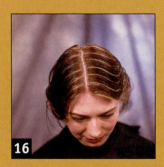

15. Continue to the front until the last foil is place.

16. In this top view, you can see where the foils were placed. They were processed to a pale yellow. Note the alternation of light and dark.

17. Apply haircolor glaze over the highlights. This will add tone and shine to the natural color, and tone the highlights. The target color is an amber light blonde. Mix 1 oz. of 10RO Lightest Red-Orange Blonde with 1 oz. of 10R Lightest Golden Blonde and 2 oz. of demi-permanent developer. Outline all four sections of the head.

18. Apply glaze all over the head in a base-to-ends fashion.

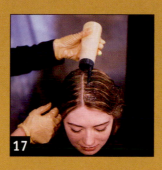
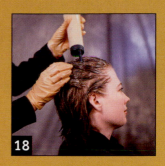

19. Work the color into the hair to make sure it is completely saturated. Process for 10 minutes.

20. The finished look shows beautiful golden amber highlights all over the head. Discuss home maintenance with the client.

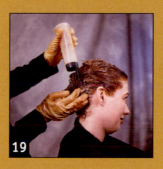
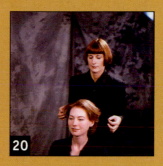

21. The finished look is dynamic, sophisticated, and glamorous. Some of the best color work is the most natural and this understated yet glorious color that accentuates the overall style is a fine example of this.

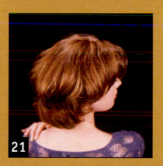

VARIATION— PANEL HIGHLIGHTS

In this service, you will create a dramatic highlight effect throughout the top portion of the head, featuring wider bands of highlights.

APPLY

ON DVD ▶

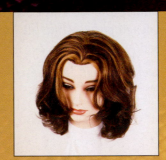

PROCEDURE

1. Part out the top portion of the head from the middle of the eyebrows. Starting at the crown area, take a fine slice and put it into a foil.

2. Apply the product to the strand and fold the foil.

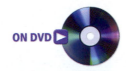

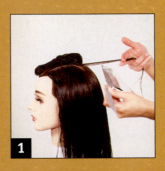

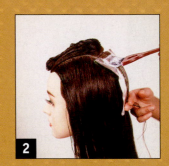

3. Without taking a subsection of hair to remain unlightened as in previous technicals, take another slice and place it right behind the first one. This will make for thick highlights that process effectively. Here you can see two foils back to back. Part out a 1" subsection to be left unlightened between the foils and work neatly and efficiently. Clip the hair not being worked on out of the way.

4. Part off a fine slice from the top of the section released.

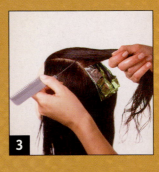

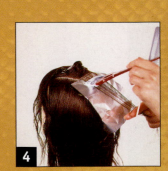

5. Place it into the foil and apply the product.

6. Continue working to the front of the head using the procedure as outlined—two fine slices foiled right next to each other with a 1" subsection unlightened in between the foils.

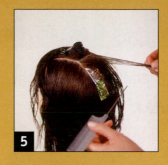 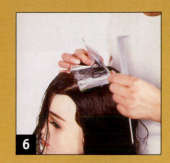

7. Take a 1" subsection in between the foils.

8. You can see the two foil packets back to back, with 1" subsection in between.

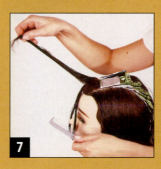 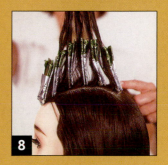

9. This look creates dramatic highlighted pieces of hair on the top surface of the head.

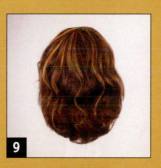

VARIATION—CHUNKY FRONT PIECES

This is an easy way to add dramatic light pieces to the fringe area.

APPLY

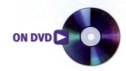
ON DVD ▶

PROCEDURE

1. Take a 1″ subsection from the front hairline. Take a fine slice, place it into the foil and apply product.
2. Double fold the foil.

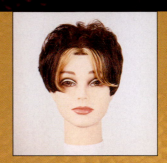

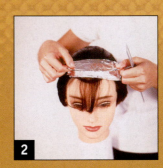
1

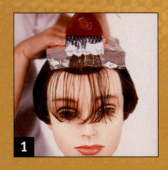
2

3. Take the next slice of hair back to back with the first one, and place it onto the foil.

4. Continue placing foils to the front hairline. Fold the edges of the foil back to secure.

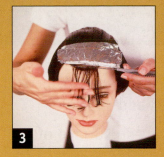

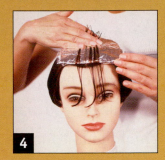

5. Here is the finished view of foils.

6. This look creates bold highlights in the front fringe area. This is a definite statement for a more progressive look. You can also tone the hair if desired.

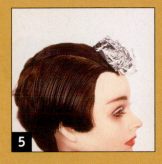

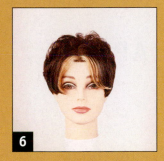

VARIATION—BALAYAGE TECHNIQUES FOR ADDING SUBTLE HIGHLIGHTS

The word *balayage* means "to paint." Whenever you want to add subtle highlights to make the top surface of the hair sparkle, this is an easy, fun way to do so. The product you will use here is a powdered lightener.

APPLY

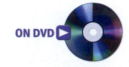

PROCEDURE

1. Apply the powdered lightener to a tail comb or color brush and lightly paint the product down the strand.

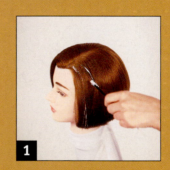

1

2. Work downward diagonally around the entire head.

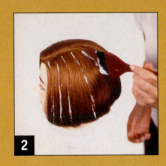

3. Once the balayage technique is completed, let it process for 10 to 15 minutes. Rinse and apply a color-enhancement formula over the highlighted hair if desired.

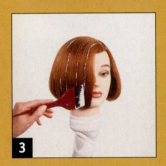

4. Haircolor highlights strategically placed are a dramatic, yet quick and practical addition.

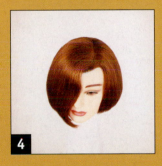

CREATE

Apply this technique to different hair lengths, colors, and cuts for almost endless possibilities.

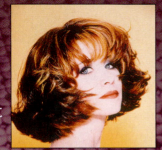
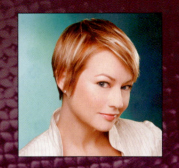
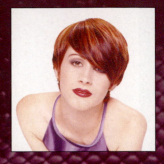
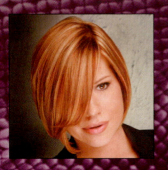
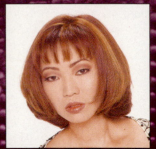

CHEMICAL TEXTURE SERVICES

PART 2

BRICKLAY ROLL TECHNIQUE

OVERVIEW

Clients today desire "instant gratification" with their hairstyles. This includes the results of their texture services—a client wants to comb through or run her fingers through her hair and have it fall into place effortlessly.

In this section you will explore using the bricklay setting technique to set the entire head. This setting pattern will be one of the most frequently used in the salon. The flow of movement in the finished result looks natural and can be easily maintained by your client. Hair flows with no discernible splits between rows. The bricklay setting pattern will expand and enhance voluminous movement and dimension. The tool diameters used here will create a firm, resilient curl pattern.

The backswept direction off the face opens up and keeps hair from falling in the face. It moves hair back and up against the natural fall of gravity, creating desirable volume. The setting pattern for this set involves beginning at the front

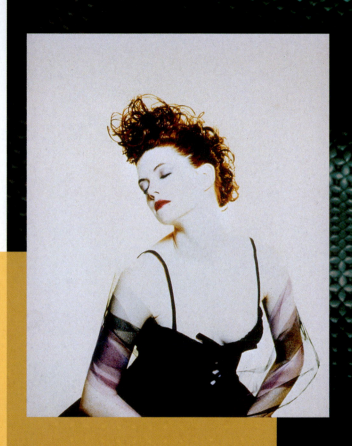

forehead area with the first tool placed. This serves as the starting point for all subsequent partings through the top and sides to parallel each other. At the crown, horizontal partings are taken that continue down to the nape.

APPLY

ON DVD ▶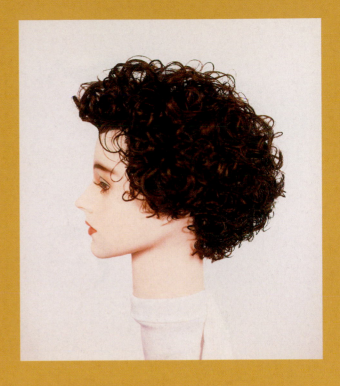

After your consultation, drape the client, shampoo and cut the hair according to the directions for the Low Graduation cut.

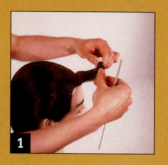

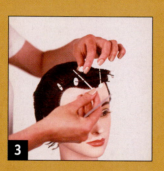

PROCEDURE

1. Begin the set at the front hairline area by parting out a base area that is the length and width of the longer rod you are using. Comb and distribute the hair 45 degrees above the center of the base area. Apply a double end paper wrap. Roll from the ends to the base to position the rod on the base area.

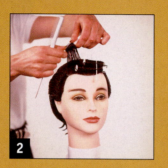

2. In the row directly behind your first rod, take base partings that allow for two midlength rods to be offset from the center of the first rod.

3. Insert picks underneath the bands to alleviate pressure on the hair.

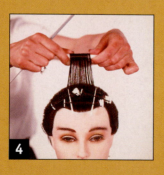

4. Before you set the next row, study the area to be set. Adjust the rod length as needed to accommodate this area. Now begin the next row by positioning a rod at the center of the spot where the two rods met in the previous row.

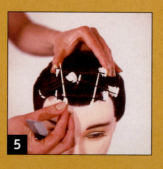

5. The pattern you see here is the one you will use throughout the entire set.

6. Continue to part out rows that radiate around the curve of the head, extending around and down toward the side hairline area. Maintain precision parting out, distribution, and rolling of hair strands to create the bricklay pattern. Secure the rods and insert picks, either as you go or when you are finished.

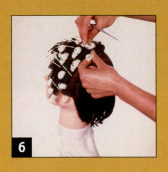

7. At the crown area of the set, instead of curving rows around the front hairline, take rows that work around the back of the head in a horizontal fashion. Continue with the bricklay pattern. As you work from row to row, adjust the length of the rod to fit into the area you are working on.

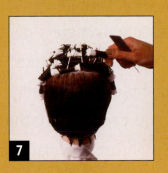

8. When you reach the occipital area, change to a smaller rod to create more curl definition and support. When lengths become quite short, change your end paper technique. Fold single end paper in half, and bookend wrap, to control and smooth the ends.

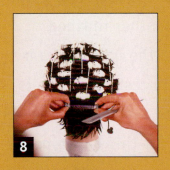

9. Complete the bricklay wave set in the nape area. As you move toward the perimeter area, progress to a one-diameter base size with the rod positioned half off-base.

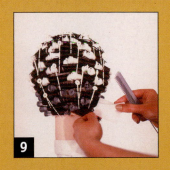

10. The highly active texture and support in this design fully expands the shape, providing a tremendous amount of volume. The backsweep of hair from the face is highly prized by clients who want to make a textural statement but still easily maintain their styles.

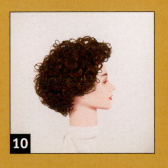

BRICKLAY-ROLL TECHNIQUE I

OVERVIEW

This highly textured style provides the ultimate volume and definition of the cut shape. Alternating texture diameters gives a very natural curl. This type of texture can be diffused naturally or air formed with a round brush; you can also dry the texture in naturally, then use thermal styling tools, such as hot rollers or curling irons, to create a smoother finished effect. Before waving the hair, perform a porosity and elasticity test to gauge its condition. The waving system used will be specifically selected for this hair type—a fine texture, normal density, and color treated.

APPLY

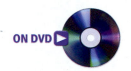 ON DVD

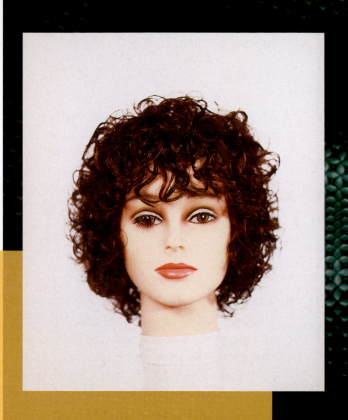

PROCEDURE

1. In the finished wave set, two different diameter rods alternate in a directional movement swept back off the face. To add to the naturalness and flow of movement, each base part is weaved or zigzagged throughout the set. Begin setting at the front forehead area by zigzagging the tail end of your comb along the scalp area to part out the first base area.

2. Note the base parting.

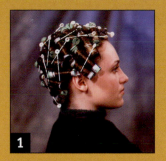
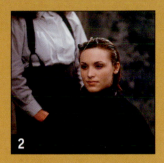

3. Roll the first section on the larger rod to position on base. The bricklay pattern will begin from this rod position.

4. Continue to roll row after row with the bricklay pattern. Zigzag the base partings and alternate rod diameter from row to row. At the crown, begin rolling half off-base. Note the zigzag base parting.

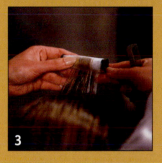
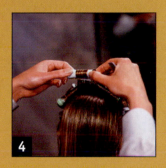

5. Continue rolling directionally toward the nape area. At the perimeter hairline area, roll the larger rod upward in an indentation technique.

6. The rods are directionally rolled back off the face and rolled diagonally at the sides, shifting direction at the crown to begin rolling horizontally downward. Apply the appropriate liquid styling tool, in this case a liquid gel, and diffuse hair for a natural finish.

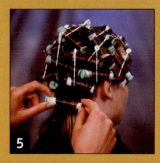
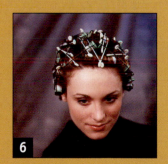

OVERVIEW

In this design, the bricklay set will add texture to the classic, heavily layered shape. The symmetry of the cut shape is quite conducive to this low-maintenance, easy-care, easy-wear style. All the hair around the front hairline is directed toward the face. The lengths framing the face soften the facial features. Texture flows directionally from the crown area, providing voluminous movement and dimension.

APPLY

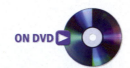

ON DVD ▶

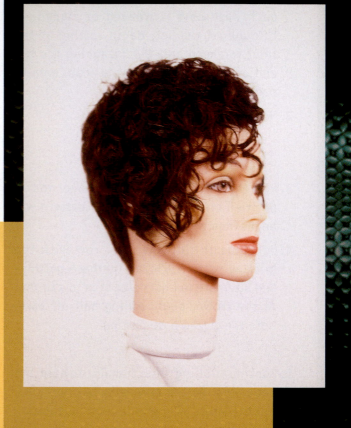

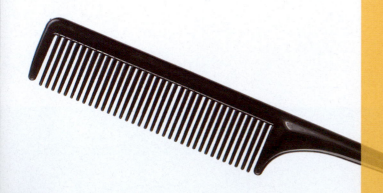

PROCEDURE

1. In the finished wave set, all rods radiate from the natural growth direction in the crown area. Direct all rods in the front area of the set forward in a bricklay pattern; all rods through the back area of the head flow from the crown downward in a bricklay pattern.

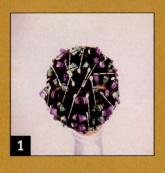

2. Distribute the hair into front and back sections by parting out from the central crown area to behind the top of the ear on each side of the head. In the center crown area, which is directed forward, part out a base area to the length and width of the larger rod you will be using for this set.

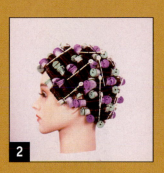

3. Divide the first sections using a weaving technique. Move the tail end of the comb to alternate between strands of hair. Comb one of the woven portions toward the back area; you will roll it, along with the back area of the head, later. The other woven portion will be rolled forward.

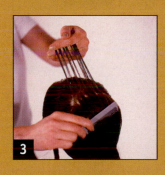

4. Distribute this strand of hair 45 degrees above the center of the base, and roll it to the base, to create a one-diameter on-base rod position. This will provide lift in this area.

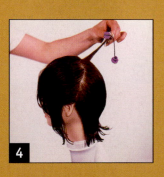

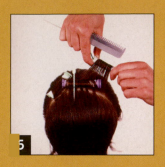 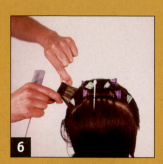

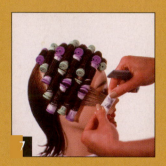 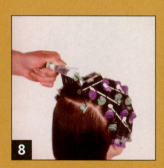

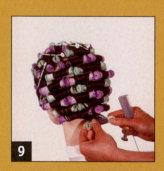 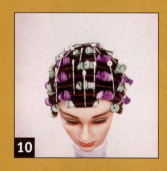

5. Begin to alternate rod sizes in the next row; adjust your rod lengths as needed to fit within the rows. Roll all rods in the front area forward, toward the face. In the third row, return to the central area to begin rolling from this area outward.

6. Work toward the outer side of the row on either side of the centrally positioned rod. Continue to alternate between the two rod sizes from row to row.

7. Complete the bricklay set in the front area by working to the front hairline. Adjust rod sizes and lengths to allow for the hairline lengths around the face. When the front area is complete, move to the crown area.

8. Part out a base area the length and width of the smaller of your two rods. Distribute the hair 45 degrees above the center of the base area for rolling. This will create a one-diameter on-base rod position, maximizing the volume in this area. Roll lengths back and down from the crown area.

9. Alternate rod sizes from row to row through the back area. Finish the bricklay setting technique at the nape area.

10. In this alternate view of the finished bricklay set, note how all rods directionally flow from the crown area outward toward the perimeter hairline area. Use picks to lift the bands away from the rods.

CREATE

Apply this technique to different hair lengths, colors, and cuts for almost endless possibilities.

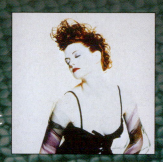 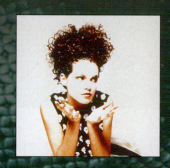 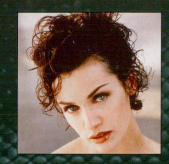

OVERVIEW

This classic texture set waves the hair into a formation that provides the client with great versatility. Whether diffused for soft natural movement that accentuates the dimension of the style, or blow-dried smooth for voluminous style support, this set pattern is an important one to add to your repertoire of skills.

This set pattern encircles the curved contour of the head. Within panels, roll the hair directionally. These panels surround a central panel, which you part out from the front forehead area to the central nape. Then divide the remaining

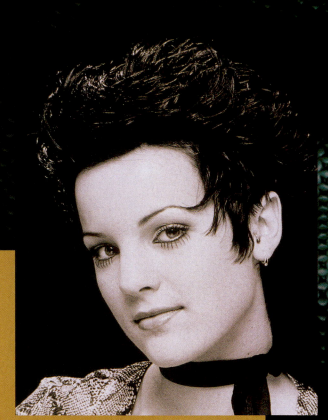

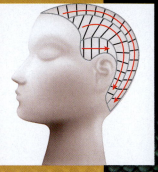

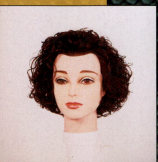

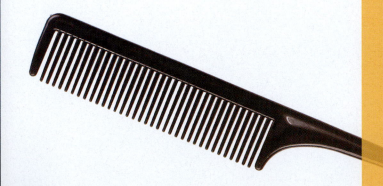

profile (side) areas to reflect the directional movement that you are looking for in this area. Your rods should progress in size from larger in the interior, where the longest lengths are, to medium size around the perimeter, where more support is desired.

This set pattern is versatile enough to be used on virtually any cut shape—blunt, graduated, or layered. In this demonstration, the pattern accentuates the shape of the diagonal back blunt cut.

APPLY

ON DVD ▶

After your consultation, drape the client, then shampoo and cut the hair according to the directions for the DIAGONAL BACK BLUNT CUT.

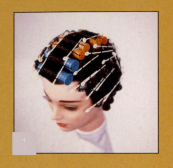

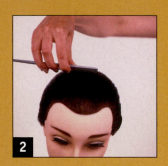

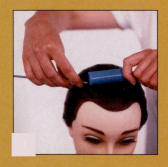

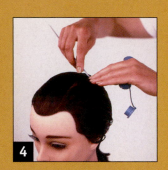

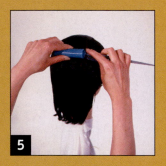

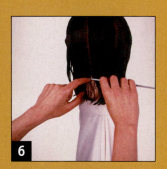

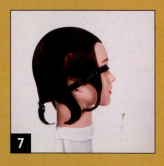

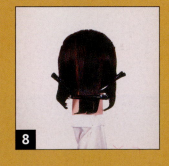

PROCEDURE

1. Here is the finished wave set. The texture tools curve to fit the shape of the head as they move away from the face. A central panel that is the width of the longest rod extends from the center forehead area to the center nape. On each side of the head, the partings curve from the temple area to the outside nape area.

2. Prepare to set this pattern by directing all lengths back away from the face. Comb and distribute the hair smoothly.

3. Beginning at the front hairline area, part out a panel as wide as the rod you have chosen. Position the rod at the center top area to provide a guide for parting off the panel on each side. Take the parting along one side from the forehead area to the crown.

4. Part out the other side of the panel to the crown. Separate the hair gently on each side of the part; try to maintain the original backward hair distribution.

5. Continue this procedure throughout the back area of the head. Position the rod centrally and then part from the crown to the nape.

6. Part out along the other side of the rod length to complete the central back panel.

7. Use this same technique for sectioning out panels on each side. Place rods at an angle at the temple area to measure panel width, because the desired direction moves down and back through this area.

8. Keep in mind that this set is being done on a mannequin head, however; every client you work on will have differences in head shape, head size, hairlines, and growth patterns.

9. Use the rod to measure and section out the base area to a one-diameter base size. You will use extra-large-diameter rods through the center top to match the longer lengths of hair there. Progress to large-diameter rods around the exterior of the shape, which has shorter lengths.

10. After parting across with the tail end of your comb, lift the tail end up and back through the hair as shown. Try not to disturb the surrounding hair.

11. Comb the hair smoothly 45 degrees above the center of the base. Apply double end papers to the ends of the hair. Roll the lengths from the ends to base area.

12. The rod will position itself on its base area given the angle of rolling. This technique is used to create strong base lift, hence volume, through the top area.

13. You can insert picks while you work through the set. After the set is complete, the picks will support the rods while keeping the band away from the hair. Continue to roll lengths through the top area using the same rolling angle.

14. At the lower crown area, you will make a change in both rod size and base control. Comb the hair straight out from the center of the base area in preparation for rolling. The rod will position itself half off-base, which will slightly diminish the amount of base lift.

15. Comb the hair straight out from the base and continue to roll lengths straight toward the center nape.

16. Use the rod to measure and diagonally part out the base area. Roll the rod so that it positions itself at a diagonal.

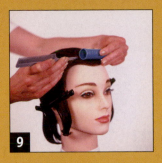

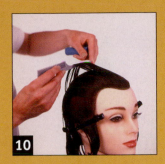

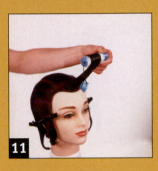

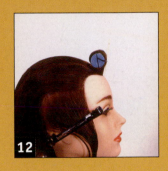

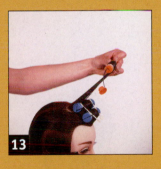

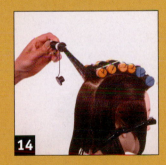

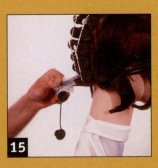

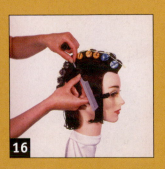

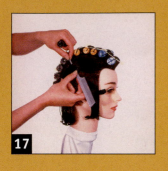

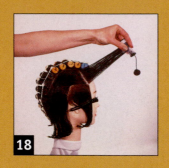

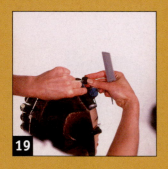

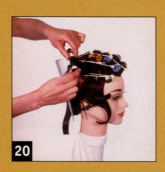

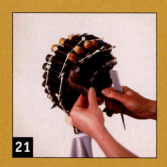

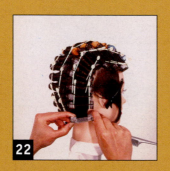

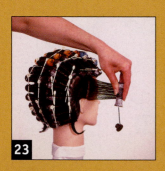

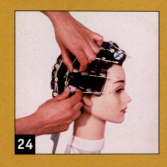

17. After parting, lift the tail end of your comb up and back through the hair. Try not to disturb the surrounding hair in the panel.

18. Comb the hair 45 degrees diagonally above the center of the base area. Using this technique in the side areas around the front hairline gives extra base support and lift.

19. Roll the rod to the base area and fasten. Assess the hairline strength, density, and growth patterns on your client's head to determine the most appropriate base control. Fine hair with less integrity around the front hairline, for instance, will require less tension; you might also want to use a half off-base control.

20. As you round the curve of the head toward the back area, change your base control. Hold the hair straight out for rolling and position the rod half off-base. Note the diagonal rod positioning.

21. As you turn toward the nape area, your base sections will be slightly wider along the outside edge of the panel; this will allow you to turn from the diagonal back position to a downward direction. On the mannequin, taking one or two base sections around this curve should be enough.

22. Continue to roll lengths through to the nape area. Use shorter rods in this panel to adapt to its width.

23. At the area above the ears, section hair vertically beginning at the front hairline area. Direct lengths diagonally downward from the center of the base area and then roll to position the rod on base.

24. Roll all rods vertically and in a backward direction through this area for the client who prefers to wear her hair off her face.

25, 26. Here is the finished wave set again, seen from two different views. Observe the rod size and positioning from the top interior area toward the exterior. Note the directional movement within the panel areas—the hair goes back and off the face in a movement that echoes the curve of the head.

27, 28. The textural expression of movement and dimension in this design enhance the cut shape beautifully! And this texture is versatile enough to allow for a wide variety of style changes.

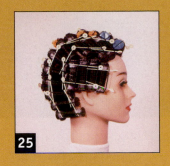

25

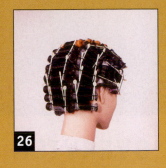

26

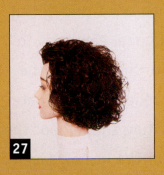

27

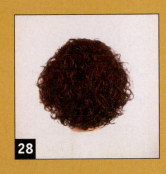

28

CREATE

Apply this technique to different lengths, colors, and cuts for almost endless possibilities.

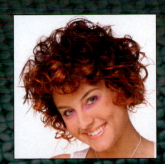

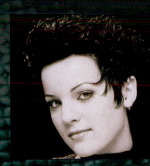

CURVATURE SET

OVERVIEW

In this wrap, the panels used throughout the head have a directional emphasis to them—they contour to the curve of the head. This curvature panel setting creates a seamless flow of texture throughout the lengths to complement the heavily layered cut. The flow of hair is very natural as well as extremely manageable for the client.

Essentially, the curvature panel setting takes into account the desired style lines, and how the client will wear her hair, making styling easier for her. However, the style has built-in versatility, given the flow of one panel into the next, particularly through the interior. In addition, the area framing the face is set within a curvature motion. Contrast this to block setting, in which lines are rigidly set in a downward directional throughout the exterior of the set.

The movement created throughout the interior allows for the hair to blend beautifully from the front forehead area to the back.

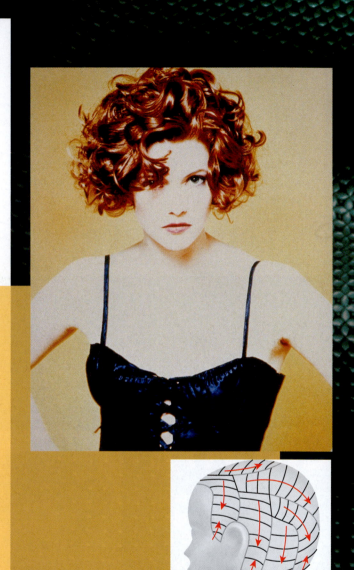

APPLY

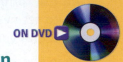

ON DVD ▶

After your consultation, drape the client, then shampoo and cut the hair according to the directions for the heavy layer cut.

PROCEDURE

1 The finished curvature panel set, incorporates a directional backward movement off the face within panels that curve around the head. Rod sizes alternate within the panels. Roll the rods for volume until you reach the perimeter of each panel, where you use an indentation application to create a more closely contoured effect.

2. Panels flow one into the next throughout the central region of the head, from front hairline to nape.

3. Begin by sectioning out the curvature panels throughout the entire head. Comb the hair in the direction that the hair will move, then section out individual panels to match the length of the rod you will use. Begin this procedure at the front hairline area off of the side part area.

4. Alternate from side to side as you section out the panels. Here is the finished sectioning pattern from the back.

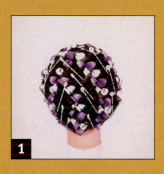

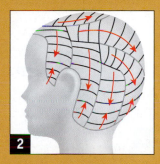

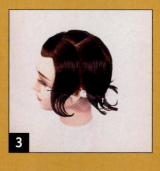

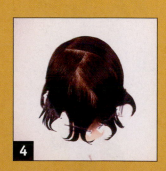

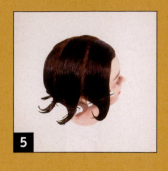

5

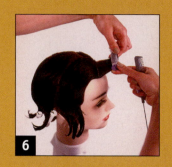

6

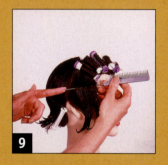

7

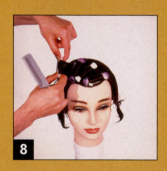

8

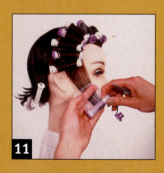

9

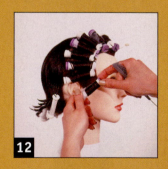

10

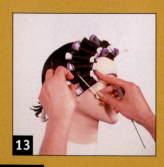

11

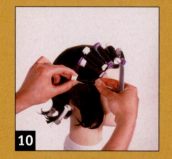

12

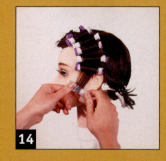

13

14

5. Pre-sectioning of the curvature panels you will use to roll this texture set will allow you to set neatly and in clear directions—it will give you a road map or blueprint.

6. Begin the curvature setting at the front hairline area, next to the side parting. Part out a one-diameter base size and roll the rod to the on-base position.

7. Stabilize your rods as needed while you roll.

8. As you work through the panel, continue parting base sections that are expanded around the outside area of the panel, the area farthest away from the face. The base areas should remain one diameter around the front hairline area. When you reach the crest area working over the curve of the head, distribute the hair straight out from the base area to position the rod half off-base.

9. Note how the base is being parted out of the panel so as not to disturb the surrounding hair. Lift it out and around in a curve.

10. Alternate rod diameters as you work toward the perimeter.

11. When you reach the last rod to be rolled, comb the hair flat at the base and position the rod in preparation for rolling up and away.

12. Roll the rod up and toward the base while keeping the base area flat. In this set, use the larger diameter rod to roll perimeter lengths in the indentation technique. This will maintain closely contoured movement within this area.

13. Because of the flat base you get with an upward-rolled rod, insert the pick in an upward direction.

14. Move to the other side of the head and set the panel around the hairline on the lighter side of the part, using the same technique.

15. Move to the panel behind and next to the first one you set. Roll rods with an on-base rod control throughout the top area of the head; change to a half off-base control toward the exterior, until the perimeter area. Set the last two rods in each panel in the indentation technique to accentuate the effect.

16. Add a pick after rolling; the upward directed rod requires support.

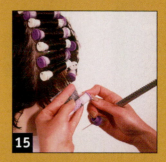
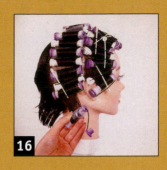

17. Return to the panel on the opposite side of the head and roll for volume using the same technique alternating rod sizes within the panel. Here is the back of the head with two panels left to roll.

18. Roll all rods for volume in this panel until you reach the perimeter area, where you roll the rods upward.

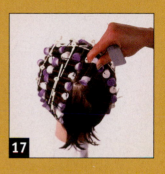
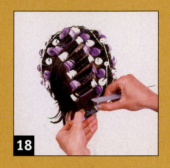

19. Insert picks to secure the rods and ease any band tension on the hair.

20. Complete the last panel. Note that the directional movement within this panel should remain consistent with the pattern you have already established. The directional movement throughout the back flows around and contours to the perimeter hairline area.

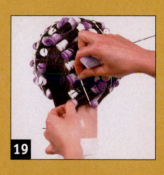
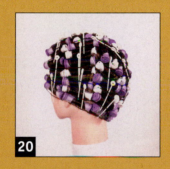

21. Note how all panels fit the curvature of the head, and how the rod alternation is consistent within the panels up to the perimeter rod. The panels all connect and blend into surrounding panels.

22. Here the finished texture has been diffused dry—this is the most representative finish of the wave set. Note the flicked-out areas around the perimeter, which combine and harmonize with the mix of voluminous texture throughout the interior of the style.

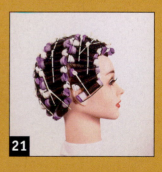
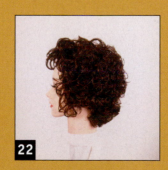

CREATE

Apply this technique to
different lengths, colors,
and cuts for almost
endless possibilities.

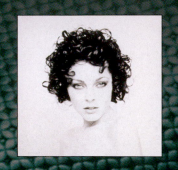 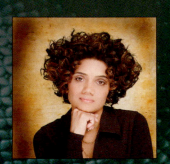 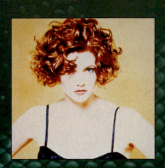

CURVATURE/BRICKLAY COMBINATION

OVERVIEW

This set is a quick and easy way to introduce texture and body. Curvature movement around the face, with a rolled bricklay pattern through the rest of the set down to the occipital area, creates a carefree, versatile texture. A variety of style changes is possible—the hair can be dried naturally, blow-dried with a round brush, molded, or wet set. In this demonstration, a vented roller is used. The roller is vented to allow thorough rinsing of solutions from the hair.

APPLY

ON DVD ▶

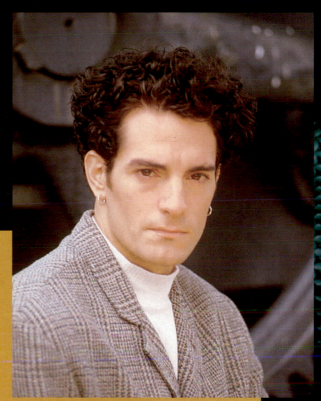

After your consultation, drape the client, then shampoo and cut the hair according to the directions for the horizontal graduation cut.

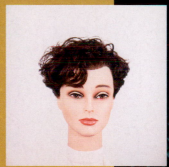

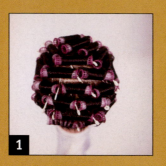

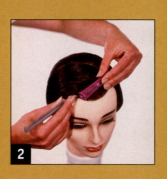

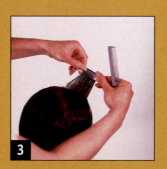

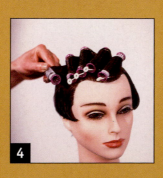

PROCEDURE

1. To create the finished wave set, set the lengths in a bricklay pattern from the top apex area of the head toward the occipital area, until hair becomes too short to roll on a large-diameter rod.

2. Begin at the top front hairline, placing the rod as a measurement for a one-diameter base size. Part out through the molded panel. Lift up and around so as not to disturb the remainder of the molded section. The base will be approximately one diameter in width at the front hairline area and then expanded at the outer back edge of the panel.

3. Holding the hair at a 45-degree angle above the center of the base area, roll to position the rod on the base.

4. As you continue, take base sections with an outside area that is slightly wider than the inside area. As you start to travel over the curved crest area of the head, take the hair sections straight out from the base. This will create a slightly diminished base volume as you move toward the shorter perimeter lengths.

5. At the area above the ear, weave the section as shown. Roll the top of the woven section to rest on the base. Try to keep a large, open wave pattern here, to harmonize with unwaved perimeter lengths. If the length here does not roll onto the rod you have been using, do the weave on the section just above it. Repeat this on the other side.

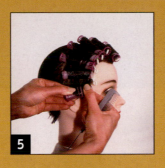

6. Bricklay through the crown and back area. When you reach the shorter perimeter lengths, again use the weave technique to roll the last row of rods.

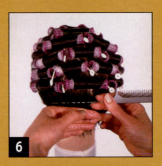

7. Roll the rods in this last row along the top of the woven section. Pick to secure.

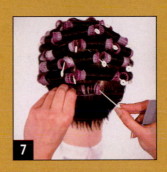

8. The finished wave set.

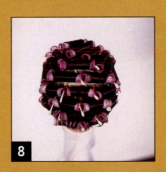

9. In the finished style, note how the texture accentuates the shape while giving directional support and contour to the hair lengths, for ease of styling.

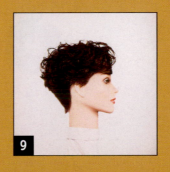

VARIATION—PARTIAL BRICKLAY II

OVERVIEW

A very commercial and desirable approach to texture for many clients could be called "texture à la carte." This is the positioning of texture in only those areas where the client needs or wants support, lift, and movement. In this short layered shape, for instance, texture was introduced into the crown area only. We have elected to use a bricklay pattern within a diamond shape that reflects and complements the lines of the haircut.

Begin the procedure by studying the natural growth patterns through the crown area and determining the most appropriate beginning and ending areas for your set. Then distribute the hair around the curved region of the head from a pivotal area at the top of the crown, where the movement is to begin.

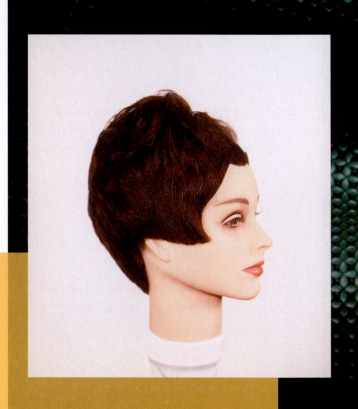

APPLY

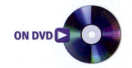

ON DVD ▶

PROCEDURE

1. Create a zigzag base part in preparation for rolling.

2. You will use very large diameter rods in this set to blend smoothly into the surrounding unwaved lengths of hair. Roll the first rod within the diamond shape. Continue to part out and roll rods from row to row using the bricklay pattern.

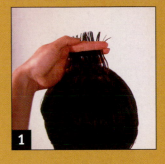

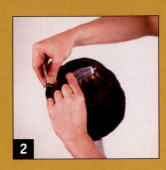

3. Continue the bricklay setting pattern within a diamond shape. The set diminishes at the upper occipital area.

4. Note the finished wave set through the entire crown area within the diamond shape. All base partings have been zigzagged. The set area is surrounded with cotton to protect the surrounding hair (unwaved) from the waving solution. You can apply a conditioning cream to the hair outlining the set area before you place the cotton, to provide extra protection.

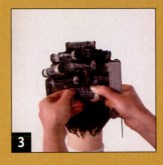

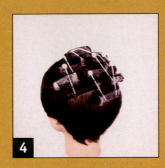

5. This finished style is a perfect example of "texture à la carte." The partial crown volume balances the style, adapting to the client's face and head shape. It is a very contemporary approach to waving the hair, and it allows you to discuss texture with clients who would not consider a full wave set.

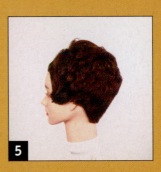

CREATE

Apply this technique to different hair lengths, colors, and cuts for almost endless possibilities.

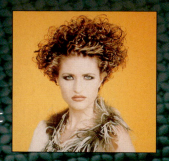
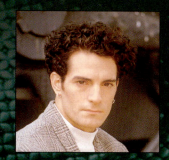
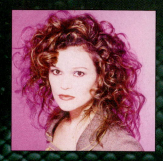

BRICKLAY ROLL AND SPIRAL TECHNIQUE

OVERVIEW

The bricklay pattern is a classic technique for arranging or setting the tools in position for waving. It creates a smooth flow of movement because base partings are offset from row to row. In this design, we transform the shoulder-length Horizontal Blunt cut to create luxurious wave patterns, movement, and dimension.

The rolling and spiral techniques are fundamental for creating a wide variety of textural effects. The techniques remain the same whether the pattern of application is within direction, curvature, or straight movements.

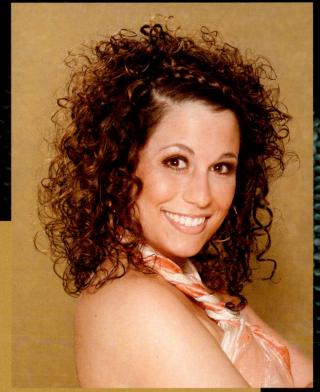

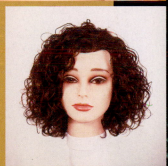

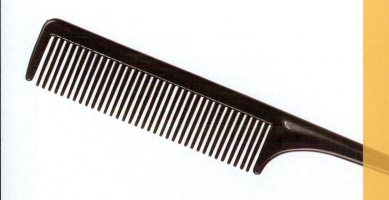

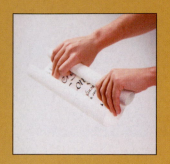
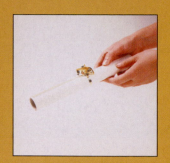
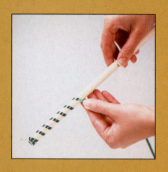
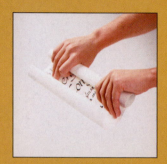

The rolling technique involves rotating the tool to wrap the hair evenly around it (similar to the way you would roll a diploma or scroll). Spread the hair evenly along the tool and roll smoothly toward the base. This creates a strong undulation. The spiral technique involves winding a strand of hair along a tool from one end to the other (similar to winding a ribbon around a dowel). This creates natural-looking elongated texture.

APPLY

ON DVD ▶

After your consultation, drape the client, then shampoo and cut the hair according to the directions for the Horizontal Blunt cut.

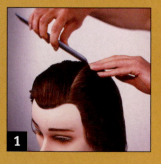
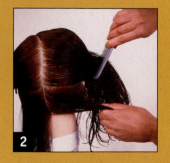

PROCEDURE

1. Begin the procedure of setting by sectioning the hair off through the natural side part, curving towards the center crown.
2. Start at the center crown and part down the center back vertically. Part horizontally from the occipital area to the center back of the ear on both sides to subdivide the nape area.

3. Begin at the top center area of the nape section by placing the rod and parting out to the length and width of the rod (a one-diameter base size).

4. Comb the hair straight out from the base parting. Place two end papers over the ends in preparation for rolling the hair smoothly. This is a double end paper method.

5. Position the rod at the ends and begin to roll the hair smoothly toward the base area, maintaining the hair position straight out from the base you roll.

6. Secure the band and cap across the rod when reaching the base area.

7. Continue to roll the hair lengths on either side of this center rod. Use the length of rod and amount of rods needed to complete this row.

8. Offset the rod positioning in the next row from the center top rod. This will ensure no hair splits between rows. Adjust rod length as needed to adapt for your client's head size, hair line, etc.

9. Complete the bricklay rolling technique in the nape area. Position picks through the bands. Turn the band toward the top of the rod before inserting the pick.

10. The completed nape area indicates a bricklay pattern with horizontally rolled rods.

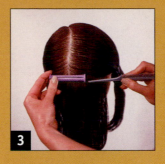

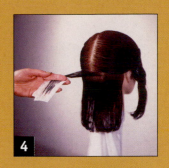

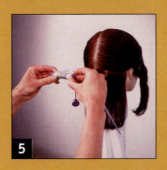

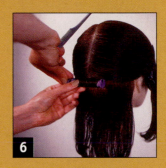

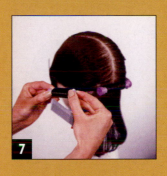

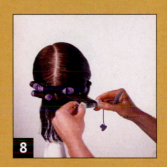

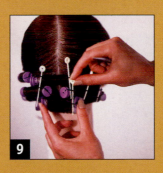

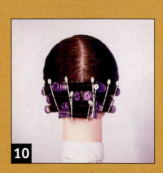

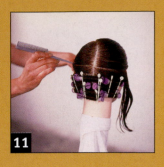

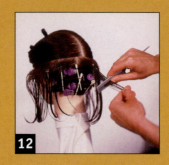

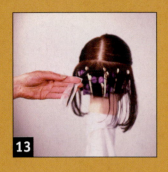

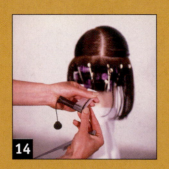

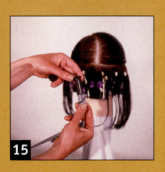

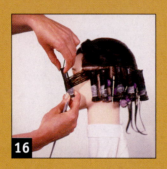

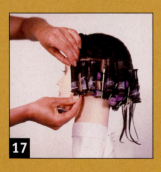

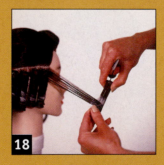

11. Part out 1"-wide subsections, for spiraling the hair onto rods vertically from center back to the front hairline. The 1" width can vary depending on the amount of base lift desired.

12. Part out base sections that are approximately the width of the rod. Comb the lengths diagonally outward from the base area in preparation for spiraling the hair.

13. Fold the end paper lengthwise over the ends.

14. Place the end of the rod at the ends of the hair and roll at least one and a half revolutions to secure the ends. Note how the end where the rod will be secured is toward the bottom.

15. With the ends secure, spiral the hair onto the rod. Secure the rod at the bottom when reaching the base area.

16. Continue to use this method of spiraling lengths onto the rod working toward the side front hairline area. Maintain consistent hair sections as spiraling.

17. Secure the rod at the bottom. Proceed to the other side of this section.

18. Follow the same procedure of spiraling along the length of the rod, maintaining a slight diagonal position.

19. Continue to divide the hair as you work upward into the 1" subsections.

20. Working around the curvature of the head, be aware of the distribution from the curve of the head. Hold the hair diagonally outward before spiraling.

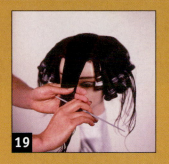
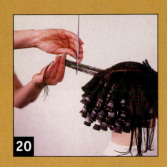

21. Secure the ends of the hair (one and a half to two revolutions) at one end of the rod, and then proceed to spiral lengths along the rod.

22. Maintain a slight diagonal on the rod as spiraling toward the base before fastening to secure.

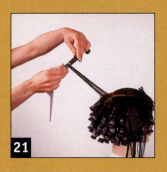
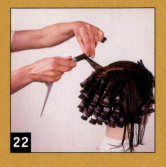

23. Fasten to secure.

24. Continue to subdivide as you work upward.

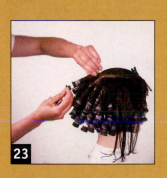
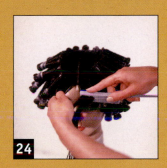

25. Note how the rod is positioned to allow for fastening along its bottom. Notice how each row of rods overlaps the previous sections.

26. Consider the possibilities! This technique may be adapted to create a wide variety of style effects. The finished texture result creates dimension and adds dynamic movement to the blunt shape of the cut.

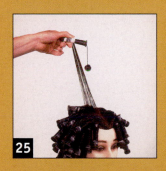
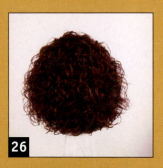

VARIATION— BRICKLAY-ROLL AND SPIRAL TECHNIQUE I

OVERVIEW

In this finished texture, a full head of sensuous ringlets creates a highly kinetic effect, truly "beauty in motion." The interesting mix of textural qualities in this style creates a very natural look that many clients will want.

APPLY

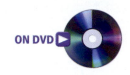

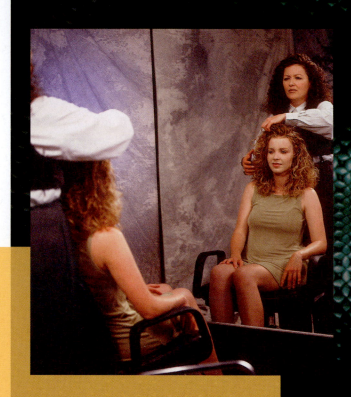

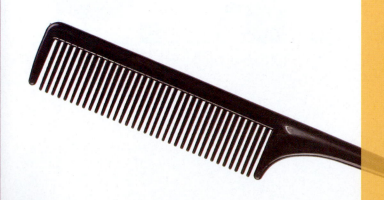

PROCEDURE

1. This client's thick, dense, long hair has never been treated chemically. For the desired style, we will spiral the hair lengths to create full explosive volume and texture with lots of movement.

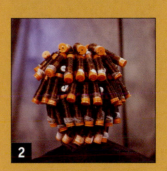

2. In the finished wave set, note the alternation between two different rod diameters, and their positioning. The white rod's diameter is smaller than the larger rod's diameter. This smaller rod is rolled horizontally throughout to alternate with panels of spiraled rods positioned vertically to add texture, strength, and definition.

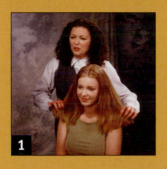

3. Spiral hair throughout the first panel in the same direction, then release the next section to be rolled, measuring this section to the diameter of the smaller rod. Beginning at the center back, distribute the hair straight out from the base area and roll horizontally from the ends to the base.

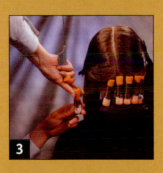

4. Fasten the rod at the base area and roll the remainder of this section horizontally. Extend the next 2" panel into the side area. All rods in this panel are spiraled and overlay the rods underneath, requiring these rods to be lifted when applying lotion to the lower rods.

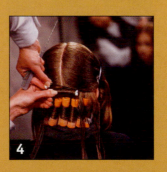

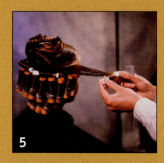

5. Continue this alternation of horizontally rolled rods with spiraled rods positioned vertically within the panels.

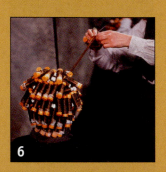

6. Take sections across the top of the head and distribute the hair up and out from the base area. Adjust the rod sizes and positions as you approach the front hairline to fit the needs of the client. In the front hairline area, roll the smaller rods forward to create more movement around the front hairline, framing the face.

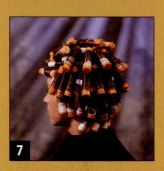

7. The completed wave set shows the alternation of rod sizes and positions. Note how the alternation in the top area of the head moves across the top, not around the curve as you did around the exterior area.

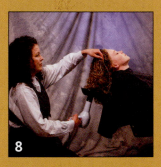

8. Apply firm-hold conditioning foam and, using a diffuser attachment, have the client drop her head back so that the hair falls freely. Gently cup the hair up into the diffuser attachment and gently massage, lift, and separate the hair as needed, but do not scrunch it.

VARIATION— BRICKLAY-ROLL AND SPIRAL TECHNIQUE II

OVERVIEW

The spiral and roll bricklay technique that was done on the longer Blunt Cut is used here on shorter lengths to create a natural springy ringlet formation. In this next style, the textural result was created on a variation of the Graduated Blunt Cut at jaw length.

APPLY

ON DVD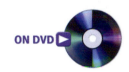

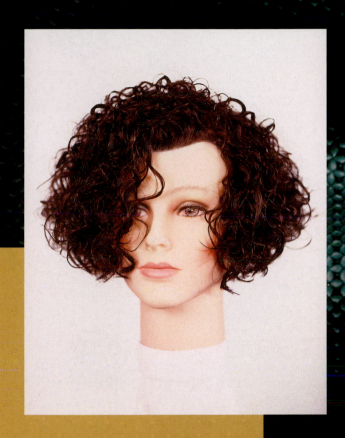

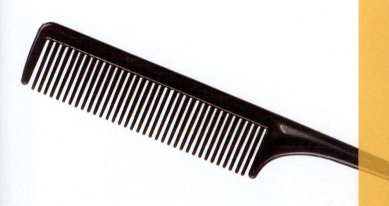

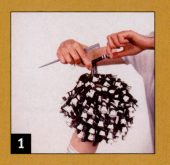

1

PROCEDURE

1. Use the same technique that was outlined earlier to progress through the set. Maintain consistency of hair distribution and rod positions as you progress through the wave set.

2. Adjust for the natural part, if required. Here, use picks to support the rods away from the forehead to clear this area for client comfort.

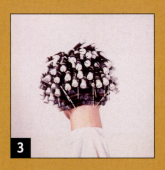

3

3. Adjust the rod size, length, and setting pattern as required for the desired result.

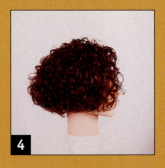

4

4. The spiral technique can be highly effective on shorter lengths, particularly blunt and graduated forms—it creates a natural ringlet effect.

VARIATION—SPIRAL BENDER TOOLS

OVERVIEW

The spiral technique is used here on the Light Layered Haircut to create enhanced volume throughout its shape. This shows the versatility of the spiral technique—which can be adapted to all lengths of hair. In this wave set, you will use soft bender rods to spiral the hair lengths. These rods come in a variety of diameters and lengths. Adjust according to the length of hair and the results you are looking for. Here, a progression of diameters is used—smaller throughout the nape area, progressing to midsize throughout the crest area, and large throughout the top.

APPLY

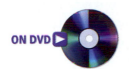

ON DVD

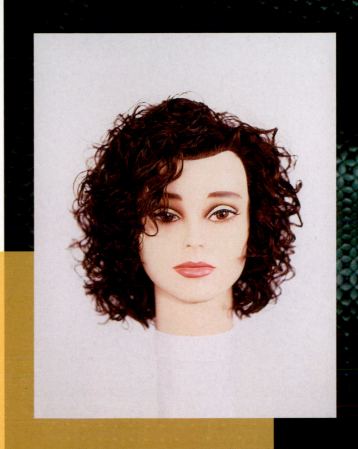

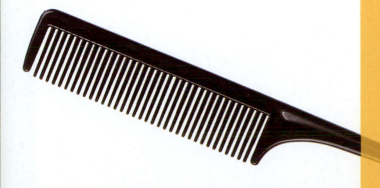

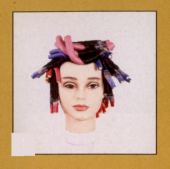

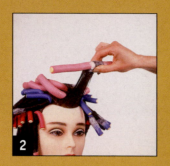

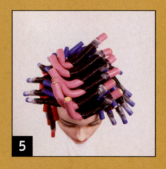

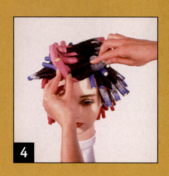

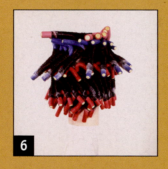

PROCEDURE

1. Take partings throughout each section on a diagonal to create a directional influence in that section. Directions alternate within each row.

2. Comb the hair lengths on a diagonal from the base area. Secure the ends of the hair at one end of the tool by revolving or rolling the ends one and a half to two turns around the rod.

3. Begin spiraling the remaining lengths of hair toward the base area.

4. Secure the tool at the base area by turning its end in the opposite direction from how you spiraled the hair.

5., 6. In the finished wave set, you can see the progression of the rod diameter sizes—smaller at the nape area, to mid-size around the crest, to larger at the top area of the head. Directions alternate from one spiraled panel to the next.

CREATE

Apply this technique to different hair lengths, colors, and cuts for almost endless possibilities.

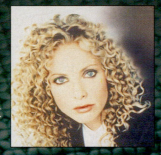
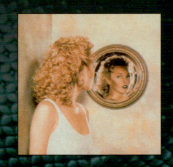
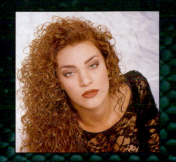

SPIRAL WITH CIRCLE TOOL

OVERVIEW

In this design you will build on your spiraling technique by using an elongated tool for extra-long lengths of hair. This allows you to work quickly and efficiently. The texture service will be done on the very long blunt shape combined with subtle long layers around the front area of the cut.

The circle tool is ideally suited to create a resilient, springy, spiral texture in long lengths of hair. This long layered shape has been set with an alternation of tools that progress in size from panel to panel. This allows more movement on the bottom lengths of hair, then progresses to a lesser, yet still firm, amount of texture through the top of the design.

APPLY

ON DVD ▶

After your consultation, drape the client, then shampoo and cut the hair according to the directions for the Horizontal Blunt cut. Notice that layers have been added on the sides.

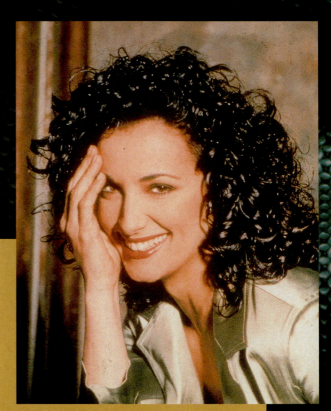

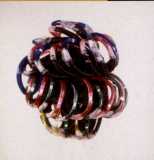

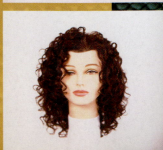

PROCEDURE

1. Here is the finished set. Bricklay the elongated, vertical base sections within each panel.

2. Begin setting in the nape area. Section out a panel approximately 2 ½" deep from ear to ear. Part out vertical base sections that are the same diameter as the rod you are using. To spiral, secure the ends of the hair, by applying a single end paper folded lengthwise, then rolling one and a half to two times to engage the ends of the rod. With the ends secured, begin to spiral along the length of the rod, working toward the base area.

3. Maintain an even tension from the ends to the base area. Secure the rod by fastening the ends together. This will be the process used throughout the head.

4. Here is the completed nape panel.

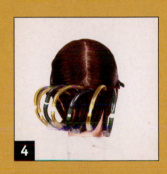

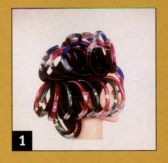

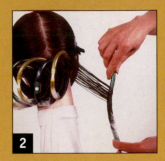

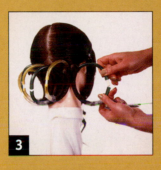

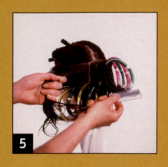

5

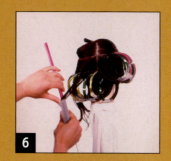

6

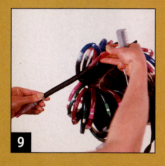

7

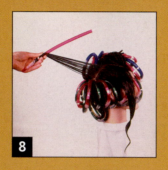

8

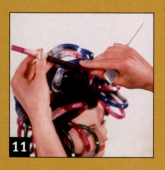

9

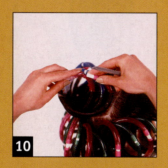

10

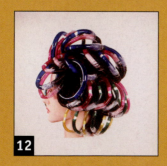

11

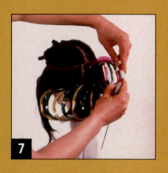

12

5. Section out the second panel above the first. Begin setting at the side opposite from where the first panel began, and move in the direction opposite the direction you established in the first panel.

6. Secure the ends of the hair by rolling them along one end of the rod one and a half to two times, and then spiral along the length of the rod. Maintain an even tension from the ends to the base area.

7. Secure the rod by fastening the ends together. Continue to work around the head.

8. Move to the panel encircling the crest of the head, and continue the same technique—but add yet another, larger rod size into the mix. It alternates with the larger of the two rods from your second panel.

9. Within this panel, work toward the opposite side, using the direction opposite that used for the previous panel. Secure the ends and spiral toward the base using even tension. Note the angle for spiraling the hair.

10. Fasten the rod and work around toward the opposite side.

11. In the very top area of the head, begin spiraling lengths from the crown area forward. Note the angle of the rod—again, this ensures smooth tension on the hair.

12. Another look at the finished set shows the progression of rod sizes in an alternating pattern from the nape area to the top of the head. The rod directions are also alternated from one panel to the next. These techniques create a natural texture that mixes textural movement and direction.

VARIATION—PIGGYBACK/ DOUBLE STACK

OVERVIEW

This is a quick way to set long internal lengths for waving. You will stack rods on top of each other, positioning two rods along each strand of hair.

APPLY

ON DVD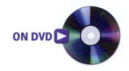

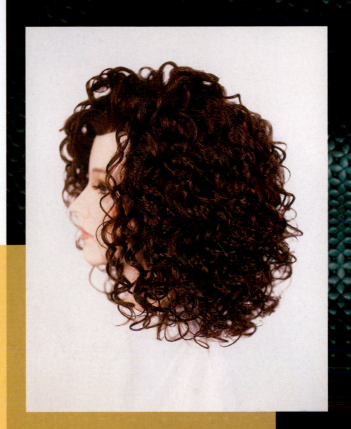

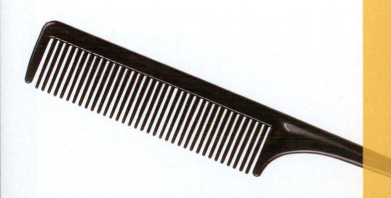

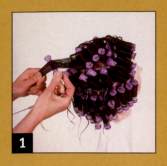

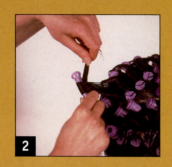

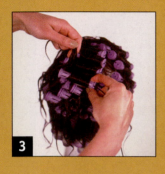

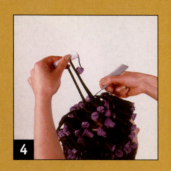

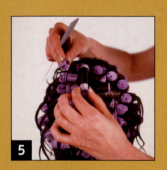

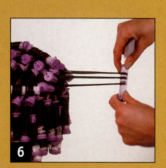

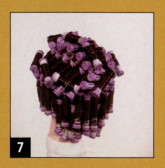

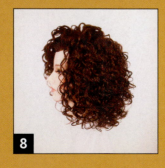

PROCEDURE

1. The perimeter of this hair has been set with a conventional spiral technique. In the interior, part out the base sections that reflect the width and diameter of the rod you are using. Place the rod at mid-strand.

2. Revolve the hair ends around the rod toward one side.

3. Now begin to roll toward the base area, letting the loose ends follow as you roll.

4. Place double end papers on the ends, and position a rod to roll from the ends toward the base area. This rod will rest on top of the rods at the base area. Use the tail end of your comb to secure the base-area rods and adjust tension before you roll.

5. Roll the rod to rest upon the rods at the base area. Maintain it straight out from the base area as you roll.

6. It is possible to join and roll three ends strands together, depending on the length of the rod you are using and the area you are working on.

7. The perimeter here was conventionally spiraled while the interior was double stacked. This technique is quite adaptable to changing diameters between the base and the end rods.

8. Use the double stack rolling technique to create voluminous texture designs on long lengths of hair.

CREATE

Apply this technique to different hair lengths, colors, and cuts for almost endless possibilities.

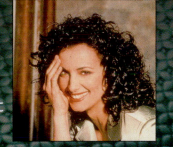
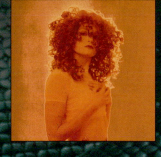
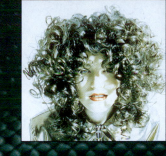
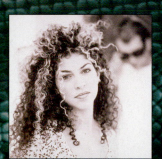
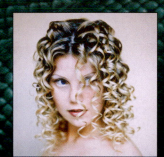

ANGULAR STACK

OVERVIEW

Setting the hair into an angular stacked pattern will allow you to expand its shape without activating the shape's outward surface. This is because the texture is placed exactly where you want it—generally underneath or along the edges of the cut shape.

The key to all texture services is embellishing the shape of the cut. The angular stack is unique in that you set the hair only to curl or wave its edges or underneath lengths. This is beneficial for a woman who prefers the texture of straight hair, but would like some measure of fullness or volume, or perhaps extra support around the edges for blow-drying or iron curling.

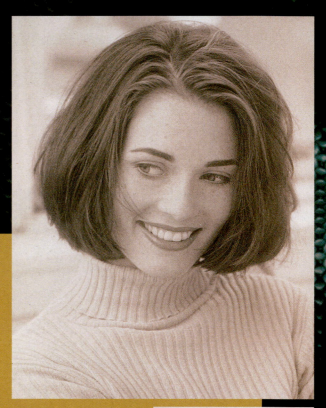

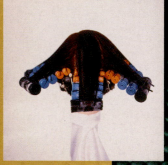

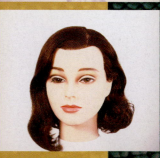

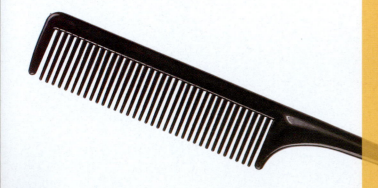

APPLY

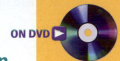

ON DVD ▶

After your consultation, drape the client, then shampoo and cut the hair according to the directions for the Diagonal Forward Blunt cut.

PROCEDURE

1. In the finished wave set, the panels are rolled to stack at an angle away from the head. Determine this angle by reaching the top length out to the stacked area and rolling it one and a half to two turns, to create a bend on the ends.

2. Bricklay the nape area first with a roll technique. Within the individual panels, the rod sizes will progress from medium to extra large.

3., 4. To create this wave set, work from the side part and section off the panels you are going to stack; they should be the width of your rod. You can measure panel widths along the bottom area, where the stack will begin. Adjust throughout the interior area according to the curve and size of your client's head. Section off the nape area from the top of the ear on each side; this will be rolled in a bricklay pattern.

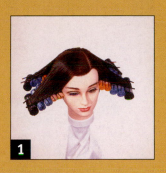

1

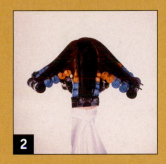

2

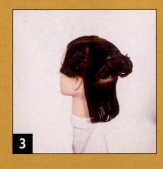

3

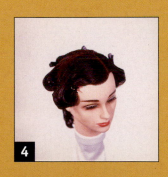

4

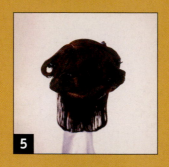

5. Panels radiate around the top curved area of the head.

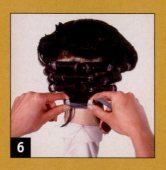

6. Roll the nape area holding the hair straight out from the base area, to create half off-base rod positioning. Adapt medium and long rods to fit into this area. When you complete the nape area, position picks to secure the rods and prevent band marks on the hair.

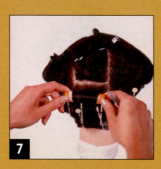

7. Begin the angular stack in the back panels. Roll a large rod from the ends to the base area, along the bottom of the panel. Use a one-diameter base size and roll with hair directed straight out from the base area, so that your rod is positioned half off-base.

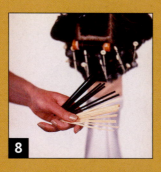

8. You can use plastic or wooden stacking sticks to angle the rods out and away from the head.

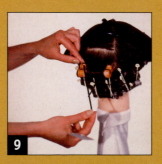

9. Before setting a panel, direct lengths from the top of the panel down toward the stack areas to gauge the angle for the stack. Roll a second rod into position, dropping it over and below the first rod you rolled. Position the sticks underneath and through the bands at the outer areas of the rod on each side.

10. Continue to work upward through the panel. Comb and distribute the hair smoothly through the positioning sticks.

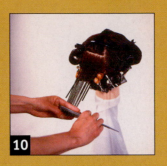

11. Position double end papers. Place a large rod (note the progression in rod size) and roll it up to rest underneath the sticks. Grasp the band and cap and stretch over the top of the sticks to secure the rod to the sticks at the predetermined angle.

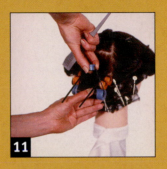

12. Continue rolling strands until all lengths are stacked at an angle along the perimeter area of the cut lengths. You will use the largest rod here to complete the progression of the texture movement.

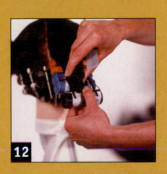

13. Use this same technique throughout all of the divided panels. During the processing and neutralizing procedure, take the client back to the shampoo bowl, and, using a gentle pressure, rinse and blot the hair. Realign the angled stacks as needed in between these parts of the service.

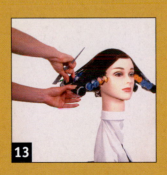

14. The finished texture provides tremendous versatility for the client who likes a smooth design, yet wants control around her perimeter weight line.

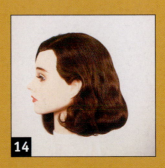

CREATE

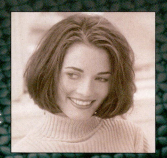

Apply this technique to different hair lengths, colors, and cuts for almost endless possibilities.

"V" FORMATION

OVERVIEW

In this design, an interesting technique creates an alternating wave movement throughout the side areas. It moves the hair back and off the face, as well as creating a very desirable volume through the interior that flows up and in toward the center.

What is unique about this set is the way tools are set in a V-formation. It creates a manageable movement and volume in this area, one that is particularly effective on shorter lengths of hair. You will use the V-formation setting on the side areas to effect an alternating wave pattern, which will flow into the freeform curl through the back area. There, you will use a bricklay setting pattern.

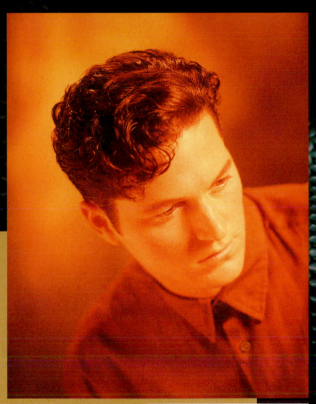

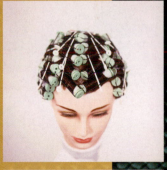

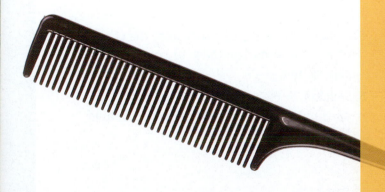

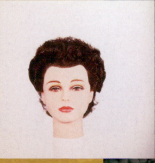

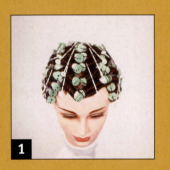

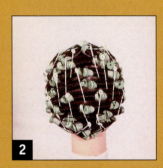

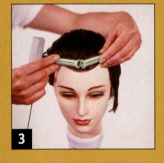

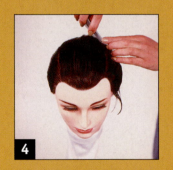

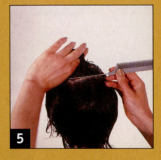

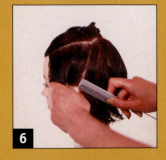

APPLY

ON DVD ▶

After your consultation, drape the client, then shampoo and cut the hair according to the directions for the Full Layers cut.

PROCEDURE

1., 2. In the finished wave set, rods are positioned through the top area in a V-formation to move the hair up and away from the front hairline. On the sides, set panels with rods positioned along opposite diagonal sections.

3. Begin by sectioning out the interior area from the sides and back. Use shorter rods positioned in a V at the front hairline to determine how wide to section off the top.

4. Section from the front hairline area back to the crown area.

5. At the crown area, section across the center of the crown horizontally, to complete the top section.

6. Section out each side by extending the parting through the crown down to behind the ear.

7. To begin setting, divide the top area vertically down the center.

8. Part out a one-diameter base size of the rod you are using (in this case, a mid-sized rod).

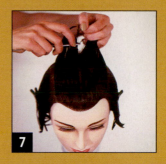

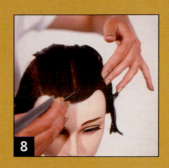

9. Roll this hair to position it on-base. This requires distributing the hair at 45 degrees above the center of the base area.

10. Roll the first rod at the hairline in the other panel. Note the V-pattern developing. This will be the procedure you will use to set rods throughout the top area-alternating back and forth between the panels as you set toward the crown area.

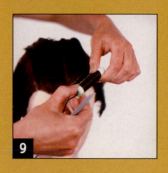

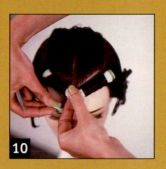

11. Continue back toward the crown area, rolling the rods within the V-formation.

12. Note the pattern developing—a herringbone pattern.

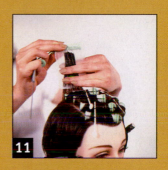

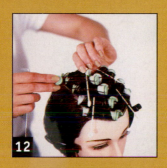

13. This is the last rod you will roll within this area. You will roll the small triangular area backward when you set the bricklay technique through the back.

14. Here is the completed top area. Adapt rod sizes and lengths as needed to accommodate your client's head size and shape.

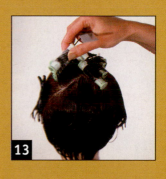

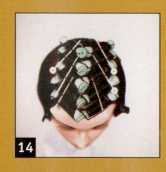

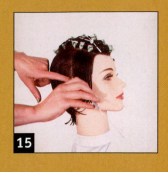

15.

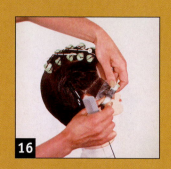

16.

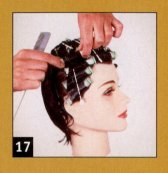

17.

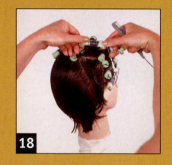

18.

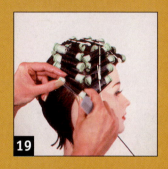

19.

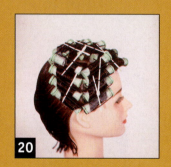

20.

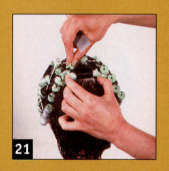

21.

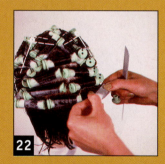

22.

15. At the sides, divide the area in half.

16. Set the direction up and back in the panel closest to the front hairline. Comb this hair upward. Part the first base area out along a diagonal as shown. Roll the rod to position it on base; you will roll all rods to position along diagonal bases through this panel.

17. Continue to part out diagonal base areas and roll rods upward.

18. In the panel directly behind the first one, roll rods downward along diagonal partings opposite those you used in the first panel at the sides. It is this change in your direction of rolling along opposing diagonal partings that will create the alternating wave patterns at the side.

19. Continue to roll the rods diagonally through the panel to above the ear.

20. This is the completed side. You can see the two panels rolled in alternating directions. Complete the other side using the same technique.

21. At the crown area, roll the first rod to begin the bricklay through the back. This first rod is positioned at the triangular area left over from the top V-formation.

22. Continue to bricklay rods throughout the back, using the volume technique. Adjust rod lengths as needed to accommodate the space.

23. When you reach the nape area, roll the rods upward in the indentation technique. Work from the outer hairline area of the nape into the center on both sides.

24. With one side complete, begin to roll the other side into the center area.

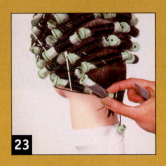
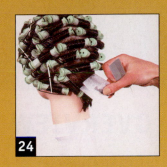

25. Adjust the diagonal parting and base positions, as well as rod lengths to fit within this area.

26. Roll all rods upward at this perimeter hairline area to create a closer contour at the base area, with a flicked-out texture on the ends.

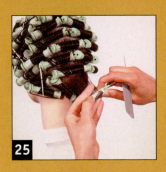
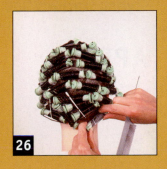

27. Here is the completed bricklay through the back area.

28. From the side view, you can see how the different areas of the set fit together.

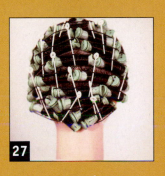
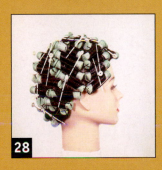

29. The finished dramatic style shows the directional movement, volume, and textural interest created through the setting technique. Here, the hair was styled by applying the appropriate styling product, then combing the hair lengths into the directional movement around the top and side areas while diffusing. The back area was diffused for full expansion and curl movement. You can also make the style and waves more dramatic and exaggerated by molding with gel—or make them soft, freeform, and voluminous using other styling techniques.

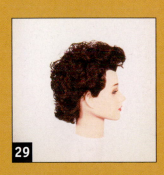

OVERVIEW

This texture set gives clients a range of styling options and great versatility.

APPLY

ON DVD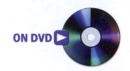

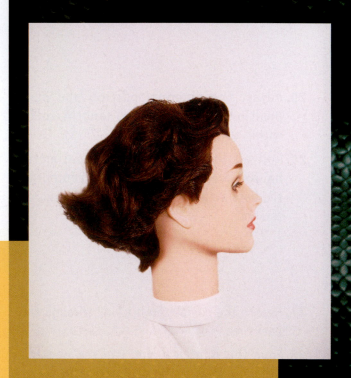

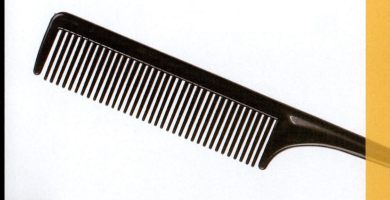

PROCEDURE

1., 2. In the finished wave set, hair is set back off the face around the front hairline, while lengths through the top and back move in alternating directions toward the nape. Do not set rollers in the nape area, where lengths are short. The texture from the rollers you set through the lower back will blend into the nape area seamlessly.

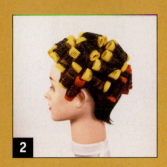
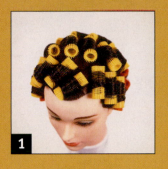

3. Section out a panel around the front hairline off a side parting. Part out a base area using a diagonal part. Take all base sections around the front hairline on a diagonal, to direct hair back off the face. Roll the hair to position on-base, maximizing base lift.

4. The on-base roller position will allow the self-gripping roller to engage the hair at the base and stay in position. If needed, you can insert a clip or pick. Section out base lengths that will enable the roller to sit within its base area and not engage surrounding hair.

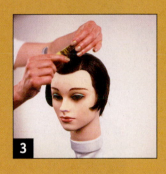
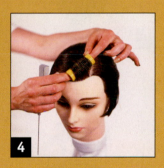

5. Continue to take diagonal partings that parallel each other as you work through the panel around the front hairline. Control the ends of the hair and roll smoothly toward the base.

6. At the area above the ear, change to a roller that is one size smaller than used in the previous panel in order to accommodate the lengths.

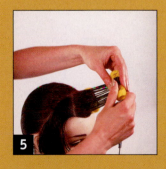
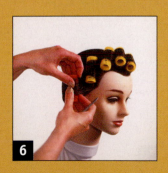

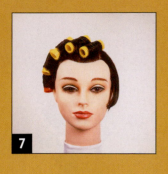

7

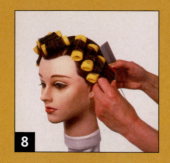

8

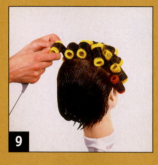

9

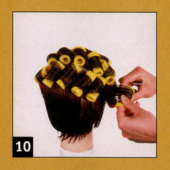

10

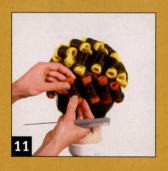

11

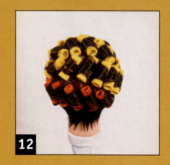

12

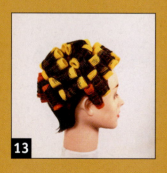

13

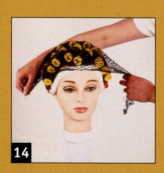

14

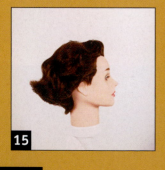

15

7. Here is the completed side off the side part. You can see that all rollers have been rolled back away from the face.

8. Set the other side using the same technique. Take diagonal partings and roll the hair back away from the face.

9. At the top area of the head, section out a panel in which you will roll the self-gripping rollers along diagonal partings. The movement from the panel at the front hairline will turn and blend into this top panel.

10. Section out the next panel across the crown area. Reverse the direction from the previous panel. Part out diagonally across the panel and roll the roller parallel to the base area.

11. Section out the next panel to travel across the occipital area. Set the rollers in the direction opposite the previous panel. Note that the diameter size is smaller through this panel to accommodate the shorter lengths.

12. Here is the completed back area. Three panels move in alternating directions from the top of the head to the nape area.

13. This profile view of the wave set shows how the directional movement around the front hairline will flow into the panels throughout the back area of the head.

14. After saturating the rollers with wave solution, apply a durable netting around the wave set to secure the tools in position before rinsing.

15. The finished style accentuates the cut shape with soft wave movement, and the texture provides the client with tremendous versatility in her styling options.

OVERVIEW

This texture service will result in soft lift and body for the client. It will also provide width and volume around the sides.

APPLY

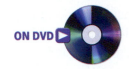

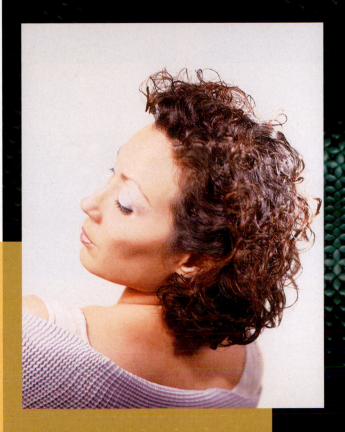

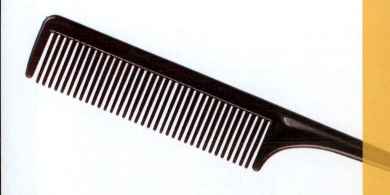

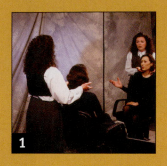

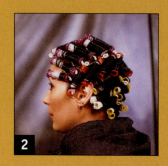

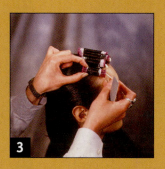

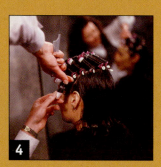

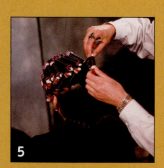

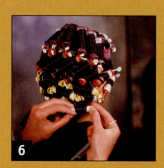

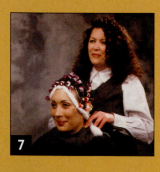

PROCEDURE

1. Discuss with the client what result she is looking for. Here, the hair designer determines that a Mid-Length Graduated cut with a directional wave is desired.

2. Begin the wave set at the fringe. Mold a C-shape, then section out a panel that is the depth of the rod. Part out the base areas by parting through the panel along a diagonal line. Roll and place rods diagonally.

3. Continue to part out diagonally through this panel, working toward the other side. Roll all rods to position half off-base parallel to the base parting.

4. Mold a C-shape all the way around the head and section out this panel, using a rod placed at an angle to measure depth. Begin setting at the temple area by parting through the panel diagonally for a one-diameter base size. Roll the rod and pick to secure. Continue throughout this panel. Switch to the opposite direction in the next panel. Change to rods one size smaller than in the previous panel.

5. Begin the bricklay pattern at the occipital area. Again, change to a smaller rod to complete the progression within the overall set.

6. Complete the nape area with the bricklay pattern. Adjust rod lengths as required to fit within the space.

7. Position a towel around the neck, with a cape over it; place another towel over the top of the cape, and clip it to secure at the neck area. Apply protective cream to the skin around the perimeter hairline area. Apply a strip of cotton around the edge of the set. Apply solution along the top and underneath areas of each rod to thoroughly saturate all hair. Replace the cotton strip around the perimeter area.

CREATE

Apply this technique to different hair lengths, colors, and cuts for almost endless possibilities.

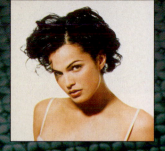
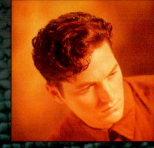

CONSULTATION AND ANALYSIS ON A VIRGIN HEAD FOR PERMANENT RELAXER

OVERVIEW

During a virgin relaxing service, you straighten hair with a relaxing product and a minimal amount of mechanical action. The manipulation is the key to a successful relaxation. When performed properly, the processing technique will yield superb results. However, when the processing has gone beyond necessity, irritation and over-processing will result. Your action should be limited to smoothing hair with the glove-covered fingers, or pressing with the back of your comb. Always wear gloves to protect you hands, and place a protective cream around your client's entire hairline. Your hands can become sensitized over a period of time to the chemicals, creating vulnerability toward contact dermatitis.

Permanent relaxers affect the hair strand by permanently rearranging the basic structure of curly hair into a straight form. Excellent products are available on the market today and come in a variety of strengths, with varying ingredients.

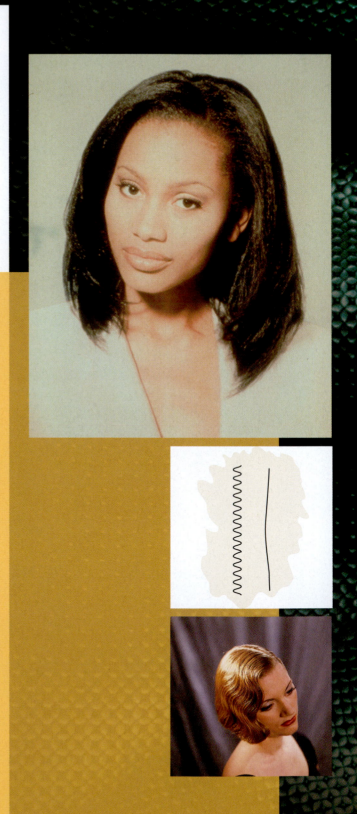

APPLY

ON DVD ▶
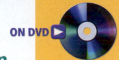

After your consultation, drape the client. The shampoo and cut will occur later in this technical.

PROCEDURE

1. Consult with your client on the style she wants.

2. Perform a strand test on various areas of the head. Move to the back crest of the head and take one hair strand.

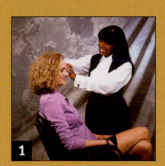

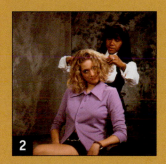

3. Hold the strand of hair firmly at the scalp and wrap it around one of your fingers to gently stretch it. If the hair stretches and does not return to its original form, or breaks, this hair has poor elasticity and should not be relaxed at this time. Run your fingers down the strand to check for porosity.

4. The strand test will tell you what condition the hair is in relative to porosity and elasticity, as well as whether it is weak, strong, dry, or oily. It will also help you determine what products to recommend.

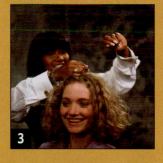

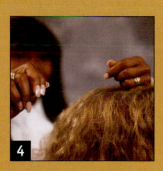

115

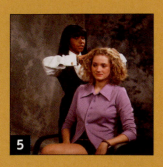

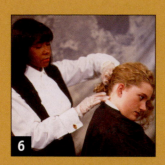

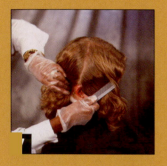

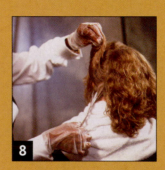

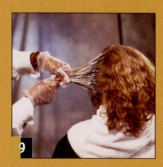

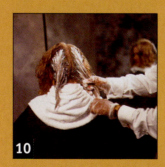

5. Evaluate the strand test. This will be the client's first relaxer, and you use a different technique to apply a new relaxer than you would to apply a touch-up.

6. Wear gloves when you apply the relaxer, and place a protective cream around the client's entire hairline.

7. Divide the client's hair into four sections, from front forehead to center nape and from ear to ear. Starting in the left back at the nape are, take 1 ½" horizontal partings.

8. Apply the relaxer with fingers about 1" to 1 ½" away from the scalp, bringing it down the entire hair strand. Work as neatly as possible in the parting, applying, and spreading the relaxer. Continue this process as you work up through this section of hair. Part out at least a couple of inches away from the scalp to prevent product from getting on the scalp.

9. After applying relaxer to the first section, take that section and bring it together, smoothing it, without allowing the relaxer to touch the scalp. Bring the smoothed hair away from the scalp.

10. In the next section, use the same technique. Applying time and initial smoothing should be done as quickly and efficiently as possible. Whether it is the first, second, or third time working through the complete head section by section, you should apply more relaxer to the area closest to the scalp as needed. Follow the manufacturer's suggested application and processing times.

11. Apply the relaxer to the third section of the hair.

12. Continue into the fourth section—proceed to part out approximately 1 ½" partings with the fingers. Then apply the relaxer through the ends.

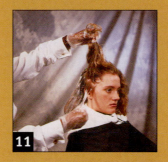
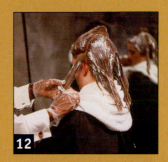

13. Complete the application technique with the relaxer.

14. Squeeze and smooth the fourth section of hair.

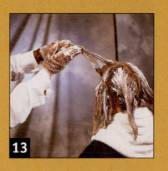
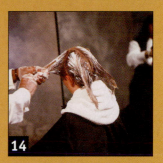

15. Move to the back nape area. With a comb, take a 1 ½" section and comb and smooth through the hair. Be as gentle as possible. Continue combing and smoothing, moving up the entire section of hair. While combing, place any excess relaxer from the comb onto the hair and continue smoothing.

16. Move to the next sections using the same technique with your comb.

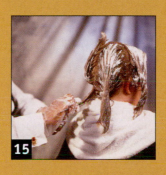
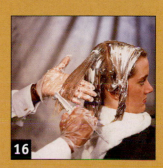

17. Use a tail comb so that you can part or section the hair with its tail end. After combing it through, there will be excess relaxer; reapply it to the hair.

18. Move onto the third section. Smoothing is very important. Smoothing utilizes the heat from the head, helping it to relax.

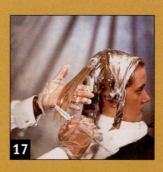
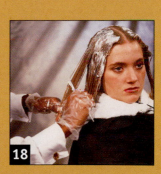

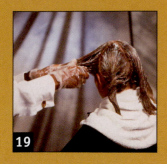

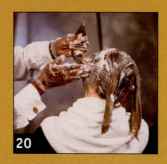

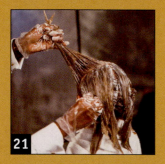

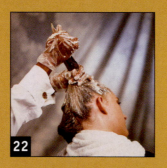

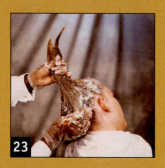

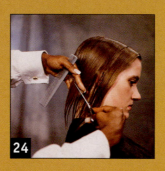

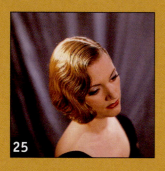

19. Work the relaxer toward the scalp and smooth through all the sections a third time.

20. Continue smoothing and working through the sections as shown.

21. The relaxer should cover the entire head as you work through the sections as shown.

22. Squeeze and smooth the sections together. Again, always reapply excess relaxer to the head.

23. Smooth and bring sections together. The relaxer is now ready to rinse out.

24. After rinsing, cut hair to the desired length and style; in this case, the Graduated Blunt cut. The hair around the front hairline is then molded into waves.

25. The finished style features soft, alternating waves framing the face to harmonize with the smooth, sleek, relaxed hair.

CREATE

Apply this technique to different hair lengths, colors, and cuts for almost endless possibilities.

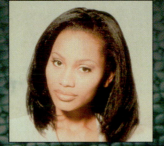
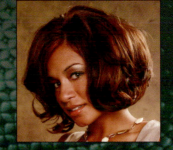
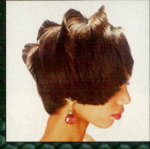

RETOUCH WITH A SODIUM HYDROXIDE RELAXER

OVERVIEW

Sodium hydroxide relaxers are generally preferred by professional stylists for the ultimate straightening. Any client who wants to reduce curl or wave is a perfect candidate for this service.

Six to eight weeks after a client has received a permanent relaxer service, new hair will have grown in, and this new growth will have the same texture characteristics as the hair before straightening. To make this new hair just as straight as the rest of the hair requires a relaxer. Applying permanent relaxer to the new growth only is called a retouch.

Here, for illustrative purposes, we will demonstrate four different methods of application, on four different parts of the head. Each method has its own unique application and processing time; each displays your presentation and technical skills in a different way. Presentation, of course, has a significant impact on your financial earnings!

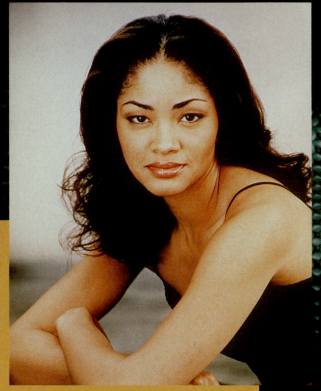

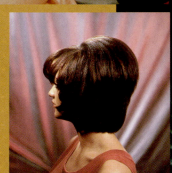

APPLY

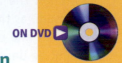 ON DVD ▶

After your consultation, drape the client. The shampoo and set will occur later in this technical.

PROCEDURE

1. Prepare your client for the relaxer service.
2. Section the hair into four parts or sections.

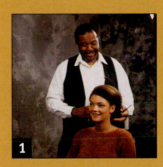

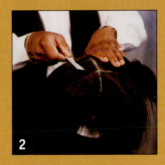

3. In the first section, you will apply relaxer from an applicator bottle. Use utility scissors to cut the tip of the applicator diagonally.

4. Put on protective gloves. Keep the applicator bottle inverted and begin outlining. Place the tip of the applicator bottle ¼" from the scalp. Continue to outline the section. Squeeze the bottle gently to flow and apply the relaxer.

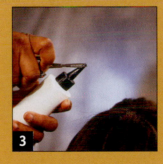

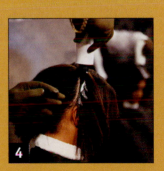

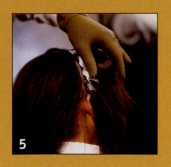

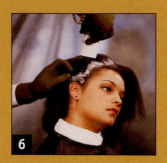

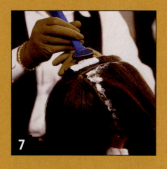

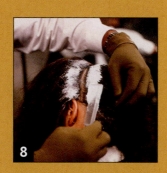

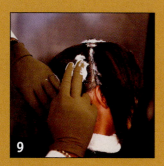

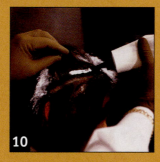

5. Use your thumb to gently spread the relaxer through the regrowth area. Do not apply pressure, as this could push relaxer through the hair and possibly onto the scalp, which might be uncomfortable for your client.

6. Continue to outline. Apply relaxer around the outer perimeter of the entire section using the same application technique, maintaining the tip of the applicator in a downward position.

7. In the second section, being the retouch process with an applicator brush. Remember to keep the product ¼" from the scalp.

8. In the third section, outline and apply relaxer for a retouch with a tail comb. Outline the outer perimeter of this section applying product ¼" away from the scalp. Note how neat and meticulous the application is.

9. In the fourth section, use a finger application technique. (Using your fingers is not as controlled; therefore, it is most often used on virgin applications of relaxer.)

10. Go back to the first section, and proceed to work through the interior. Use diagonal partings ¼" to ½" thick to apply the relaxer near the base or scalp.

11. Continue the application, working from the crown down to the hairline. Apply the relaxer, then gently smooth with your fingers, repeating this process on either side of the part as shown.

12. Continue to gently smooth the relaxer with your thumb.

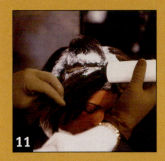 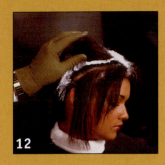

13. Finish the section. Note that using an applicator bottle for a relaxer service involves the same technique as applying tint—you will apply it ¼" from the scalp. After the product has been on the hair for approximately eight minutes, body heat should soften the relaxer and help draw it closer to the scalp.

14. Modern technology allows you to part, comb, and apply with one brush. Note that the relaxer touch-up was started in the frontal area of the head. Begin your service wherever you determine the hair to be most resistant.

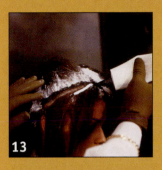 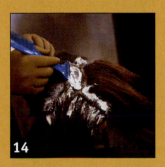

15. Work through the back section with the tail comb. Make horizontal parts, beginning at the top of the crown and progressing down to the neck area. Moving each section in an upward motion toward the crown prevents hair from resting on the neck.

16. Apply within the interior of the fourth section using horizontal partings.

17. After you have thoroughly applied the sodium hydroxide relaxer to all four sections, go back to all your partings and check the application to make sure that no product is resting on the scalp.

18. After the comb application is complete, straighten the hair by repeatedly combing with the teeth or the back of your comb and smoothing the hair. This will cause unwanted curl to straighten.

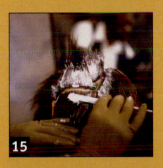 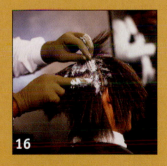

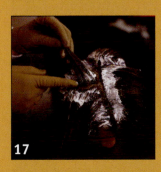 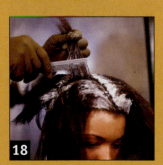

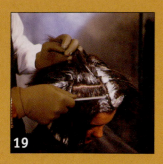

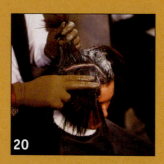

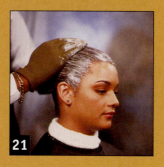

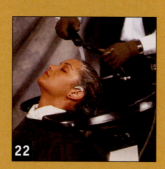

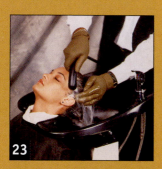

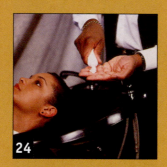

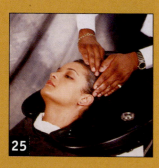

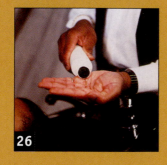

19. Using the teeth or back of your tail comb, go through all the hair, applying a small amount of pressure. This will smooth the hair, removing unwanted curl or wave. Go through the entire head of hair once or twice as required.

20. Your final comb through for a retouch involves smoothing the hair with your fingers. Work through all four sections using this technique.

21. To complete the relaxer service, work all sections together to eliminate major partings, particularly down the center top, which can occur on some clients immediately after a relaxer service. If the desired straightness was not achieved, you may need to increase the strength of the product, switch brands, or increase processing time on the client's next visit. Keep accurate records as it applies to this.

22. Adjust the bowl and the water temperature before you begin rinsing your client's hair. Start with any areas causing her discomfort, or, if there are none, with the section of hair that you applied the relaxer to first.

23. Keep the spray nozzle pointed away from the face and into the bowl.

24. When you have removed all the relaxer from the hair, the processing stops. Now the bonds of the hair are still open. This is an excellent time to use a deep penetrating treatment. Apply approximately 1 oz. onto the palms of your hands.

25. Massage the treatment into the hair shaft.

26. After you have applied the treatment, place your client's hair under a head cap for approximately 15 minutes, then rinse. Now you are ready to begin your shampoo system.

27. Use a normalizing shampoo. This will lower the pH and ensure removal of relaxer. This first shampoo is simply a deep cleansing. Second and third shampoos are recommended.

28. These shampoos may be luxurious and moisturizing for particular hair types. Rinse thoroughly after shampooing.

29. After three shampoos, apply a moisturizing conditioner or detangler and rinse out thoroughly.

30. Using a semi-permanent, vegetable-based haircolor and tint brush, paint on haircolor for highlights. Leave on until processed, then rinse.

31. Begin to blow-dry. Control tension on the hair through the angle at which you hold and maneuver your brush. This is the first step in preparing the hair for cutting.

32. The glamorous finished style! The relaxer touch up and refresher or retexturizer through the ends of the hair have harmonized the texture in this design. Color and conditioning treatments create tone, gloss, and shine.

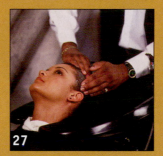

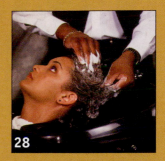

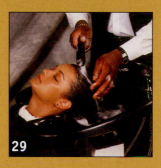

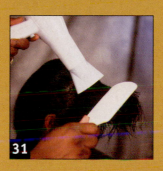

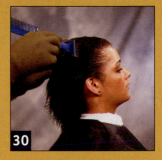

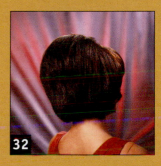

CREATE

Apply this technique to different hair lengths, colors, and cuts for almost endless possibilities.

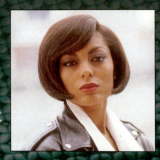 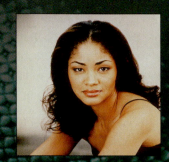